New Developments in Medicinal Chemistry
Chemistry
(Volume 2)

Edited By

Carlton Anthony Taft

Brazilian Center for Physics Research
Brazil

Co-Editor

Carlos Henrique Tomich de Paula da Silva

School of Pharmaceutical sciences of Ribeirão Preto,
University of São Paulo
Brazil

CONTENTS

CHAPTERS

FOREWORD

In modern computational medicinal chemistry, docking and virtual screening methods in drug design play important roles in aiding the pharmaceutical industries place new drugs on the market. In the first chapter of this book the authors review (homology, fragment, consensus, bioisosteric, scaffold, pharmacophore, induced fit, chemogenomics, knowledge, similarity)-based models. In addition, binding affinities, scoring functions, molecular dynamics, water and solvation, simulation of free energies, quantum mechanics/molecular mechanics, molecular fields, molecular shape and virtual screening are discussed. Some hotspots are also discussed (protein docking, stem cells, workflow pipelines, different types of ligands/targets/ interactions, (cloud/high performance/grid)-computing, post-processing, chemical libraries, confidence and the future. Docking/virtual screening programs, recent evaluations/validations/benchmarking and selected applications of various models to drug design are also reviewed.

Comprehension of binding processes, such as drug-receptor interactions, signal transduction process, and cellular recognition, are important for a better comprehension of biological functions. Medicinal Chemistry, in the path of drug discovery, has focused on studies, of the molecular interactions, which are involved in the development of severe disease states. Consequently, an accurate knowledge of the underlying protein receptor-ligand recognition events at atomic levels is important in the process of comprehension, identification and optimization of more potent drug candidates. In this sense, novel NMR spectroscopic techniques can be used as tools to gain insight into protein-protein and protein-ligand interactions in solution at the molecular level. Resonance signal of the protein or the ligand can be used to identify binding events from these experiments. In Chapter 2 the authors discuss the main NMR experimental approaches applied to identify and characterize protein-ligand binding affinity, providing a broader and better understanding of how NMR spectroscopy techniques can be employed in a drug discovery process.

Most drug candidate failures that occur during clinical trials are due to inappropriate ADMET properties. In this way, there is a major concern to identify possible ADMET failures during the early stages of drug design projects and optimize such properties in order to reduce time and costs effects. *In silico* ADMET predictions constitute several strategies that play a central role when considering the task of profiling lead compounds concerning potential ADMET failures. In Chapter 3, authors discuss the computational strategies, methods and softwares currently used to profile ADMET, which can be helpful during drug design.

Bioisosterism is a molecular modification medicinal chemistry strategy applied during drug design projects when a lead compound is available. The concept of bioisisterism is centered at the use of chemical diversity in order to optimize pharmaceutical properties of lead compounds and generate active analogs, replacing problematic substructures inside lead compounds by others with similar physicochemical properties. This can surpass the limitations observed for the original lead compound. Bioisosterism can be a useful strategy in order to optimize lead compounds searching analogs with better selectivity and synthetic accessibility, decreased toxicity, improved pharmacokinetics, enhanced solubility and metabolic stability. In Chapter 4, authors highlight the computational approaches used to identify potential bioisosters, discuss how bioisosterism can be helpful during the design of molecules with better synthetic accessibility, and review the scaffold hopping technique, a novel trend of bioisosterism application intending to identify interchangeable scaffolds among pharmaceutical interesting molecules.

This book thus attempts to convey a few selected topics stimulating the fascination of working in all the multidisciplinary areas, which overlaps knowledge of chemistry, physics, biochemistry, biology and pharmacology, describing some of the theoretical and experimental methods in Medicinal Chemistry.

Ramaswamy Sarma
State University of New York
Albany, NY
USA

PREFACE

In this book we aim to convey a few selected topics of medicinal chemistry, stimulating the fascination of working in multidisciplinary areas, which overlaps knowledge of chemistry, physics, biology, pharmacology and medicine. It contains 4 chapters, of which 3 are related to theoretical methods in medicinal chemistry and one deals with experimental/mixed methods. Docking and virtual screening methods of computational medicinal chemistry play important roles, *via* drug design, in aiding the pharmaceutical industries place new drugs on the market. In Chapter one we discuss virtual screening and comment on hotspots including (protein docking, stem cells, different types of ligands/targets/ interactions, workflow pipelines, (cloud, high-performance, grid)-computing, chemical libraries/databases, confidence, future trends). Recent evaluations, validations, benchmarking are presented. Fifty virtual screening and docking programs are summarized. Selected applications (our work over the decades) of various models of drug design discussed in the chapter are also presented. We give the basics on binding affinities, scoring functions, molecular dynamics, water and solvation, simulations of free energies, quantum mechanics/molecular mechanics, molecular fields, molecular shapes. We also review (homology, fragment, consensus, bioisosteric, scaffold, pharmacophore, induced fit, chemogenomics, knowledge, similarity)-based models.

In Chapter 2 the main NMR experimental approaches applied to identify and characterize protein-ligand binding affinity are discussed. A good knowledge of drug-receptor, signal transduction process, and cellular recognition processes are required for understanding biological functions. For drug discovery, medicinal chemistry have focused on studies of the molecular interactions which are involved in the development of disease states. Comprehension of the underlying protein receptor-ligand recognition events at atomic levels is fundamental in the process of identification and optimization of more potent drug candidates. Novel NMR spectroscopic techniques can yield insight into protein-protein and protein-ligand interactions in solution at the molecular level. Resonance signal of the protein or the ligand can be used to identify binding events from these experiments. NMR spectroscopy parameters such as chemical shifts, relaxation times, diffusion constants, NOEs and exchange can serve as measures of binding. We have attempted to provide in this chapter an overview of the NMR spectroscopy techniques employed in the drug discovery process.

In chapter 3, we discuss the computational strategies, methods and softwares currently used to profile ADMET and how they can be helpful during drug design. Many drug candidate failures during clinical trials occur due to inappropriate ADMET properties. Consequently, there is a major concern to identify possible ADMET failures during the early stages of drug design projects in order to optimize these properties and reduce time and costs. *In silico* ADMET predictions involve various strategies that play a central role when considering the task of profiling lead compounds for potential ADMET failures.

The authors highlight in chapter 4 the computational approaches used to identify potential bioisosters and discuss how bioisosterism can be helpful during the design of molecules with better synthetic accessibility. We also review the scaffold hopping technique, a novel trend of bioisosterism applications with the objective of identifying interchangeable scaffolds within pharmaceutical interesting molecules. Bioisosterism is a molecular modification medicinal chemistry strategy applied during drug design projects when a lead compound is available. The idea of this concept is centered at the use of chemical diversity in order to optimize pharmaceutical properties of lead compounds and generate active analogs, replacing problematic substructures inside lead compounds for others with similar physicochemical properties. We can thus surpass the limitations observed for the original lead compound. This strategy can be useful to optimize lead compounds searching analogs with better selectivity and synthetic accessibility, decreased toxicity, improved pharmacokinetics, enhanced solubility and metabolic stability.

Some contents of this book also reflect some of our own ideas and personal experiences, which are presented in selected topics.

Carlton A. Taft
Brazilian Center for Physics Research
Brazil

List of Contributors

Carlton A. Taft

Brazilian Center for Physics Research, Rio de Janeiro, Brazil

Carlos H. T. P. Silva

School of Pharmaceutical Sciences of Ribeirão Preto, University of São Paulo, Ribeirão Preto, Brazil

Vinícius B. Silva

Catholic University of Goiás, Goiânia, Brazil

Daniel Fábio Kawano

School of Pharmacy, Federal University of Rio Grande do Sul, Porto Alegre, Rio Grande do Sul, Brasil

Peterson de Andrade

School of Pharmaceutical Sciences of Ribeirão Preto, University of São Paulo, Ribeirão Preto, SP, Brazil

Susimaire P. Mantoani

School of Pharmaceutical Sciences of Ribeirão Preto, University of São Paulo, Ribeirão Preto, SP, Brazil

Flávio R. Pinsetta

Fellow, School of Pharmaceutical Sciences of Ribeirão Preto, University of São Paulo, Ribeirão Preto, SP, Brazil

Evandro P. Semighini

Ribeirão Preto Medical School, University of São Paulo, Ribeirão Preto, SP, Brazil

Ricardo P. Rodrigues

School of Pharmaceutical Sciences of Ribeirão Preto, University of São Paulo, Ribeirão Preto, SP, Brazil

G. R. P. Malpass

Federal Institute of Triangulo Mineiro, Ituiutaba, MG, Brazil

Jonathan Resende de Almeida

Fellow, School of Pharmaceutical Sciences of Ribeirão Preto, University of São Paulo, Ribeirão Preto, SP, Brazil

2

CHAPTER 1

Current State-of-the-art for Virtual Screening and Docking Methods

Carlton Anthony Taft[1,*] and Carlos Henrique Tomich de Paula da Silva[2]

[1]Brazilian Center for Physics Research, Rua Dr. Xavier Sigaud, 150, Urca, 22290-180, Rio de Janeiro, Brazil and [2]School of Pharmaceutical Sciences of Ribeirão Preto, University of São Paulo, Av. do Café, s/n, Monte Alegre, 14040-903, Ribeirão Preto, São Paulo, Brazil

Abstract: The current state of the art for docking and virtual screening methods in drug design have been reviewed, emphasizing their important contribution in aiding drug design and discovery. We summarize our contributions during the last decade, with proposals of novel inhibitors for Cancer, AIDS, Diabetes, Parkinson, Alzheimer and other diseases. Homology, fragment, consensus, bioisosteric, scaffold, pharmacophore, induced fit, chemogenomics and knowledge-based protocols have been described. The basics have been given for binding affinities, molecular dynamics, water and solvation, QM, QM/MM, free energy simulations, molecular shapes and fields. We also discuss virtual screening and comment on hotspots (protein docking, stem cells, workflow pipelines, different types of ligands/targets, cloud, high-performance, grid computing, chemical libraries, evaluations, benchmarks and validations). We describe the procedures of fifty programs that use the protocols reviewed.

Keywords: Binding affinity, biosiosteric, chemical libraries, chemogenomics, confidence, consensus, evaluations benchmarks, fragment, future trends, homology, induced fit, knowledge based, pharmacophore, recent virtual screening and docking programs, scaffold, similarity, validations.

INTRODUCTION

Combinatorial chemistry and high-throughput screening are among the early technologies used in the drug discovery process. With the support of computing technology/computer-aided drug design, it has been possible to lower cost and obtain higher efficiency for the drug discovery process. With *in silico* search and

***Corresponding author C. A. Taft:** Brazilian Center for Physics Research, Rua Dr. Xavier Sigaud, 150, Urca, 22290-180, Rio de Janeiro, Brazil; Tel 55-21-2141-7201; E-mail: catff@terra.com.br

design there is a reduction of time-consuming expensive experimental synthesis and characterization [1-90]. This is important when we take into consideration that an average of 12.5 years is required for development of new drugs [38]. Top pharmaceutical companies, to bring each drug to market, spend an estimated 2 billion USD.

Drug discovery aims at identifying hits and leads that interact with biological targets such as enzymes, proteins, transmembrane receptors and ion channels. Notwithstanding, there are not sufficient chemical drugs discovered yearly. This led to the introduction of virtual screening/docking techniques for faster identification of hit leads. High throughput virtual screening (HTVS) methods can filter out unpromising compounds.

The docking and screening methods are efficient but have inherent limitations. The accuracy of structures is being improved (involving flexibility, solvation, scoring functions, binding affinity prediction, configuration entropy and conformational space sampling among other issues). There are still many challenges,

In order to speed-up and guide the development of new active compounds, computer-aided drug design projects (docking, virtual screening) have been used. Effectively, chemoinformatics and computational chemistry are in full bloom due to their ability to guide the selection of new hit compounds.

Introduced in the late 1990s, virtual screening describes the identification of novel bioactive compounds using models/computational algorithms/analysis of chemical data. HTVS (high throughput virtual screening) approaches are used to find novel hit compounds that can bind to a biological target *via* analysis of large libraries of chemical structures. Pharmacophore, similarity and fingerprint scanning are among the models incorporated into HTVS.

The method is also fuelled by increasing available high-quality crystallographic structures as well as experimental protein-ligand interactions data. Extremely useful is the screening of large databases of reveals. These are already existing molecular databases whereas the hit compounds can be purchased directly for experimental testing. HTVS studies can however be challenging if there is need to properly prepare million compounds databases. Currently, many of such curated databases have been adequately designed and are available for research.

Each chemical compound in the library used in HTVS is at, in principle, a possible pose. The compounds can be sequentially docked at the protein (Target). The molecules docked with the lowest free energies of interactions are ranked in the list and considered as potential 'hits' to be possible subjects to further experimental assays. Virtual Screening programs typically consists of algorithms that search the space available to candidate molecules and a function representing a measure of binding affinity. The minimization process yields solutions for active molecules in accordance with experiment and separate active/inactive compounds.

When we speak of docking, we typically refer in general to a computational technique which places in the receptor (macromolecular target) a small ligand (molecule) and determines the binding affinity as well. The main components of a receptor-ligand structure *in silico* are a) docking (orientation and conformational sampling constrained by the binding site of the receptor) b) scoring, *i.e.* for a molecule the best ligand orientation, conformation and translation (pose). If a ligand database is docked, scoring functions are used to rank the best order of ligands. A successful docking should accurately predict the binding affinity as well as the pose.

Before starting on project, it is necessary to assess the docking, virtual screening setup, *via* literature or actually performing it to determine if the choice of program, scoring functions, and techniques for receptor and ligand flexibility are validated. There may be difficulties in positioning low-resolution structures. There may be an absence of alternative ligand structures (protonation, tautomeric states, and orientation and conformation compatibility with electron density). Crystal structures are important and docking quality can be strongly targeted and scoring dependent.

We can speed up finding good potential candidate drugs by using prediction methods based on theoretical computing methods and molecular modeling to determine the three-dimensional structure for new hit leads. Prediction accuracy of most programs currently still requires improvement. Some simulations determine the binding energy between ligand and receptor using relevant information of the complex (atomic radius, torsional angles, charge, Van der Waals (VDW), intermolecular hydrogen bonds as well as hydrophobicity of the contact force). Scoring functions, used to evaluate the results of docking conformations, yield three-dimensional coordinates, total energies and additional parameters.

It could be however advantageous to reduce the computation time, due to the very large size of the search space of possible conformations, with high-performance search methods. Different evaluations, benchmarks, validations, comparisons, libraries, programs and procedures are discussed throughout this chapter.

The topics discussed in this review are structure and ligand-based docking, virtual screening, homology-based, fragment-based models, consensus docking, biosisosteric replacements, scaffold hopping, pharmacophore modeling, induced fit, chemogenomic approaches, knowledge based drug discovery, binding affinity prediction, scoring functions, entropic contributions, molecular dynamics, water and solvent effects, quantum mechanics/molecular mechanics, simulation of free energies, molecular fields and shape, binding site-based methods, inverse molecular docking, chemical universe, protein docking, stem cells, virtual screening, workflow pipelines, different types of ligands/targets/interactions, cloud, high performance and grid computing, post-processing, chemical libraries, confidence and the future, description of 50 docking/screening programs, recent evaluations/validations/ benchmarking and selected applications of various models to drug design.

The authors published, during the last decade, numerous papers using the computer-aided drug design methods mentioned above and discussed in the following sections. The protocols used include docking and screening with proposals of new leads for diseases such as Cancer, Aids, Diabetes, Alzheimer, Parkinson and other diseases [1-37].

HISTORICAL

It has been more than twenty-five years to the foundation of JCAMD in 1987. Many papers have been subsequently published describing conformational analysis, QSAR, drug design, docking, homology modeling and other protocols/methods. Subsequently, an increasing number of programs has been used for diverse applications. The number/type of diseases as well as biomolecular/pharmaceutical problems have also steadily increased, yielding successes and doubts/claims/aspirations.

Computer technology and user-friendly software are key players in this impressive scientific and technological growth. The software makes a complex science available to novices as well as experts. Computation is today an intrinsic part of biomolecular and pharmaceutical research.

However, as we read the yearly comparisons, benchmarks, evaluations and review publications, we realize that we have not completely achieved our goals. There is still much more work ahead.

With the support of some of the first computer applications for drug design [42-90], *i.e.* (GENOA [49], DYLOMMS [50], ALADDIN [46], CAVEAT [47] early concepts/innovative techniques for the interactions between ligand and receptor were developed, *i.e.* DOCK [62], CoMFA [63], MCSS [61], GRID [51], yielding computer applications to scientists for automated drug design. The early interaction models still provide framework for recent molecular design algorithms.

LEGEND [52,53], GROW [69], LUDI [54,55] and GrowMol [66] were among some of the early key players in the 1990's. For ligand and structure based methods there are innovative procedures and strong renewal of interest in this research field, which combines multiple scientific disciplines. Current key players include Glide (Schrodinger LLC), Gold (Cambridge Crystallographic Data Center Cambridge) and Discovery Studio (Accelrys Software) among others.

Scoring, sampling and synthetic accessibility have long been the main scientific challenges for *de novo* drug design. It was argued in the early 1990s that given a target receptor it should be feasible to use algorithmic connection of small molecular fragments to model a potential ligand. This molecule should exhibit desired electrostatic and structural complementarity with the receptor [69].

Starting with peptide-mimetics, navigation in chemical space has evolved considerably into procedures including Markov chains, product enumeration, deterministic combinatorial approaches, stochastic sampling by evolutionary algorithms, simulated annealing, particle swarms, *etc*....). The field has also benefited from parallel developments in computer science and engineering yielding sophisticated tools. These include visualization of multi-objective compound optimization progress, online structure-activity landscape modeling and observation of convergence and design runs.

One of the first structure-based *de novo* design studies was published in 1976 [81]. Early methods relied on static X-ray spectroscopy that imposed pharmacophoric and structural constraints. Ligand and target flexibility, for example, were not favored. In 1995, the computer designed carbonic anhydrase inhibitor dorzolamide drug was first introduced leading a number of following successful cases [41].

Current design tools allow for molecular flexibility with a corresponding increase in CPU requirements. From a technical point of view GPU computing, cloud computing and other distributed hardware solutions will sustain progress in this research area. It is also noteworthy that chemical understanding is essential for computer-based tools that should incorporate as much medicinal chemistry knowledge as possible in the quest for drug discovery.

One of the great remaining challenges is activity and polypharmacology predictions. We are also still far from being able to make reliable estimates of entropic contributions to ligand-receptor complex formation. Innovative concept and approaches are required. There has also been complementarity between scoring concepts and machine learning models. Kernel-based regression models and artificial neural networks have the adaptability and speed for calculation of new data without need for explicit energy computation. The machine-learning paradigm may offer temporary solutions, *i.e.* target-specific and knowledge-based models. Chemical similarity is used already in scaffold-hopping. Bioisosteric replacements are used in solving scoring problems in contrast to global energy computation.

Combination of flexible pocket models, shape and pharmacophore matching (hydrogen bridges, solvent molecules among others) may contribute to progress for receptor-based drug design *via* ligand adaptation. This should help avoid, to a certain degree, extensive usage of ligand poses [42-90].

Molecular docking and high-throughput virtual screening should certainly continue playing increasingly important roles in the coming decades.

HOMOLOGY MODELING

High-quality 3-D structures of the protein target are important for ligand and high-throughput docking (HTD) in the drug design and discovery process. There is a continuous increase in the already large number of proteins available in the Protein Data Band (PDB). Despite this increase, numerous important drug targets do not have 3-d structures. As an example of this exception, we can include membrane proteins with their crystallization difficulties.

This makes it interesting to validate *in silico* homology modeling tools for said proteins. Correctly modeling the binding site could be the only alternative to obtain reliable structural models for the drug lead discovery processes. This would yield an important increase of already available structures in the PDB. It would also further consolidate homology models in structure-based virtual screening [91-149].

Homology or comparative modeling is the process of generating a structural model of a target protein from a known template structure. Homologous proteins evolve from a common ancestor. Due to mutations they can be however dissimilar. Sequence similarity can be less preserved than structural similarity. In order to maintain function, structure is typically more conserved than sequence. In regions close to the surface (loop regions) we observe the most pronounced dissimilarities. In these regions we can even find changes in the physicochemical properties of the side chains. There are less frequent changes for residues in the interior of the proteins. Highly conserved are the center of the proteins (common core of residues) and the main elements of the secondary structure. Although less accurate than high-resolution experimental methods, homology modeling can be helpful in the drug discovery process.

Using amino acid sequences (with information from other homologous structures), homology modeling is able to generate protein structural models. These can be built, taking into consideration similar structural stretches, and extrapolating features from the known homologous structures. If multiple structures are available such as template structures (basis), the procedure can be better performed. The process involves identifying structural templates, sequence alignment, modeling of structurally conserved regions, loop modeling, side chain modeling, model optimization and model validation.

The first step is to search for proteins with known 3d structures. These should be related to the target-protein (target sequence). Function similarity, structural knowledge, evolutionary correlation and expression by the same group of genes should be taken into consideration.

Since sequences of amino acids of proteins of unknown structures can be obtained, sequence similarity is often used to search for homologous proteins. In this approach, a number of requirements are necessary to determine the degree of sequence identity (construction of target structure model). It is necessary to have alignment with respect to one or more sequences of known 3D structures as well as prediction of the secondary structures that the amino acids of the target sequence will assume.

The first task is to search for proteins with known 3d structures that could be used as templates for modeling the unknown structure. They should correlate with the target protein. The Basic Local Alignment Search Tool is a useful homology software. It searches the sequence database (aligns the query sequence with each sequence in the database). It uses an heuristic algorithm to search for high scoring of sequence alignments. Specific tools are used to assess the degree of similarity between fragments of the sequences (local alignment). This is to identify, from a biological/structural point of view, important similarities. PDB and other databases can be used. Algorithms for sequence similarity searches can be applied

Once the template structures have been selected, one proceeds to align the target with the template sequences. If the percentage identity between compared sequences is high, the correct alignment should proceed. However, in the cases of low sequence identity, the correct alignment is difficult. The schemes use score pairs of all aligned residues. For example, alignment of pairs of identical/similar residues gets higher scores than dissimilar pairs. Scoring schemes includes chemical similarity, observed substitution scoring and genetic codes.

During sequence alignment there is structural alignment of equivalent residues. This includes active site regions and secondary structure elements. Gaps (insertions and deletions often present in loop regions) can be determined in both target and template structures. More efficient multiple alignment of multiple structures can also be performed whereas various sequences are compared at once.

In the third step, regarding the modeling of structurally conserved regions, we note the following. The homology approach is based on the fact that there are nearly identical families (in their 3d structures) that corresponds to regions in the proteins (inner cores). Here we can find differences in peptide chain topology which could yield significant effects on protein structure. After alignment, modeling of similar regions in the target can be done.

The core of the model can be built from equivalent aligned residues of the templates using conserved secondary structure elements present in the template structures and selecting sections from the template structures (based on an estimation of the likelihood of similarity of local environments for individual amino acids). As the number of structural templates increase, the assignment of structural conserved regions becomes more important. There should be a careful examination (superposition) to identify the more relevant regions. This is important to validate the sequence alignment.

In the fourth step regarding loop modeling, we note that in these regions occurs the most important structural differences. There are typically gaps in the alignment between model and template sequences. In the model, these gaps are related to deletions. In in the template sequence these gaps are related to insertions. Although not straightforward to predict, these changes can be limited to loop and turn regions.

Energy-based and knowledge-based are major procedures for loop modeling protocols. In the energy-based method an energy function is used to classify the quality of the loops generated (*ab initio* fold prediction). In order to select the best loop conformation, molecular dynamics, for example, can be used to minimize the energy function. A guide to model loop regions in the knowledge-based approach would be, for example, a segment of equivalent length in a homologous protein. The conformation should be the same for loops that possess the same length and amino acid character allowing direct transfer of coordinates to the model structure. Loop search protocols can also be used. Loops can be retrieved as well from peptide segments in other proteins.

Regarding the fifth stage, *i.e.* side chain modeling, we note the following. Backbone conformation and features of the local environment can influence considerable the side chain orientation. Consequently, the accuracy of the backbone coordinates also influences significantly the accuracy of the side chain localization. In addition, side chains (with various degrees of freedom) can adopt various energetically allowed conformations. At high levels of sequence identity, it is sometimes simpler to just copy entirely conserved residues from the template to the model. A knowledge-based approach (rotamer libraries) can also be used to place the side chains. Rotamers can be tried and scored successfully. The key lies in the fact that certain backbone conformations strongly favors certain rotamers.

Regarding the sixth step for model optimization we indicate the following. Minimization of the model is important to relax geometric chain/close contacts and regularize angle geometry/local bonds. Minor inconsistencies and steric clashes should be removed. Energy minimization and molecular dynamics is typically used for optimization.

The last stage is the model validation. It is important to assess quality/reliability of the homology model built. The errors in the final model depend on the number of errors in the template structure. The model's errors also depend on the percentage of sequence identity. The stereochemistry quality also depends on the accuracy of the template structure. Bond torsions, planarity of peptides, bond lengths, torsions and angles can be determined and compared.

The close packing of segments of secondary structures influences the high packing densities of proteins. Interior packing can strongly influence the stability.

Consequently, examination of the location of secondary structural elements, distribution of polar and nonpolar amino acids, buried H-bond donors and acceptors, interatomic distances and surface amino acids can help determine the degree of reliability of a protein model. Chemical environment and its influence on the folding reliability of the model can also be used to assess the protein model.

Although it may not be conclusive and could be sometimes misleading, the degree of target-template sequence identity/similarity can be an indicator of the model's quality. If there is major concern to model accurately the binding site, the fact that the sequence identity is a global measure may mask the identity of the binding site area. Proper refinement at backbone and side-chain level may offset low sequence similarity in binding site areas. The performance of homology models in docking does not always correlate well with sequence similarity. Despite not being a sufficient condition, a correct sequence alignment is necessary to develop reliable models. The final target-template pairwise alignment should be improved by multiple sequence alignments.

The backbone structure of the template can be obtained from the crude model. Nonetheless, even with state-of-the-art tools, large-scale backbone displacements might be challenging. Mid-range and small displacements can be modeled by molecular dynamics, Monte Carlo based techniques and normal mode analysis-based procedures. However, this depends on the quality of the sampling and energy functions used. Consequently single structures may not define well the target-ligand complex opening space for receptor ensemble docking (RED) as a valid approach to address protein flexibility in docking procedures.

Since diverse ligands may bind to the active site, binding side receptor flexibility could be important. A good starting point can be obtained from backbone-dependent side-chain rotamer libraries as well as information of known ligands. Protein restraints obtained from previous receptor docking can be used. This is an ensemble of ligand poses to produce models with diverse side-chain orientations that is followed by local energy minimization and re-docking. Another approach is to combine experimental knowledge of ligand binding with *in silico* modeling of induced fit effects. In LSHM (ligand-steered homology model), known ligands are used to shape and optimize the binding site through (flexible ligand)-(flexible receptor) Monte Carlo-based docking which is actually an extension to homology modeling.

It is necessary to take into consideration comparisons with corresponding performance on crystal structures, enrichment factors, docking poses, availability of template structures, the docking program, the ligand library, choice of decoy library, ligand preparation, target-dependency as well as the rigid receptor approximation.

For accurate ligand-protein docking on homology models, it is necessary to model accurately the binding sites and account appropriately for receptor flexibility. *In silico* homology modeling thus appears to be a promising and cost-effective approach established in structure-based virtual screening protocols. There is still need to develop better methods in order to accurately model target-binding sites and improve refinement at the backbone and side chain levels. The adequate refinement process may offset a low target-template sequence similarity [148].

Some useful tools that have been used for homology modeling are: 1) PDB (www.pdb.org), (Database); 2) SWISS-PROT (www.ebi.ac.uk/swiss.prot), (Database); 3) BLAST (www.ncbi. nlm.nih.gov/BLAST/), (for identifying structural templates/sequence alignment); 4) Modeller (www.guitar.rockfeller.edu/modeller/ modeller.html), (for model building); 5)WHATCHECK (www.cmbi.kun.nl.swift/ whatcheck/), (for model validation).

Some authors have used docking with knowledge-based scoring functions and homology models to obtain good success rates of pose prediction [141]. Other workers have used template-target alignment methods and evolutionary distances with a set of homology models and crystals structures to produce robust docking results [143]. Another approach involves homology models with binding site optimization (induced-fit docking) which yields improved docking results [149]. Homology models can also be used for binding into a number of important receptors [91, 142-149].

FRAGMENT-BASED

FBDD (Fragment-based drug design) yields a very promising approach for optimization and discovery of lead compounds. The experimental approach is confronted with challenges and limitations. Good solubility of fragments, high quality of target protein and expensive detection equipment are required. The theoretical approach can significantly improve the success and efficiency of lead discovery and optimization. The protocol is used in parallel or independently with experimental FBDD [150-229].

The key step in drug discovery is the identification of small molecules that selectively bind to a biological target. Fragment based drug design (FBDD) constructs novel lead structures from small molecular fragments taking advantages of both random screening and structure-based drug design (SBDD).

FBDD uses fragment screening (hundreds to thousands of small low molecular weight fragments) to identify weak binders of the desired target. The hit-to-lead optimization process may involve a combination of fragment linking, fragment evolution, fragment optimization as well as fragment self-assembly.

FBDD has advantages including generation of high chemical diversity, sampling large chemical space, high hit rates and high ligand efficiency (LE = -logIC$_{50}$/number of heavy atoms). Challenges include coverage of a larger fraction of total diversity space and suitable classes of targets. It is also necessary to take more into account ligand specificity or selectivity, changes of geometries and key interactions of original fragments upon evolving into lead compounds. Future trends should include more efficiency in selecting proper linkers to bridge fragments, addition of adequate fragments and prediction of binding modes of new molecules.

The computational FBDD starts with a fragment library design, which can provide various filters, physicochemical properties, chemical diversity analysis, synthetic accessibility, solubility predictions and fragment information. The fragment screening stage can include pre-filtering of fragment library (fragment docking), virtual hit identification (fragment docking), and hit expansion (substructure or similarity search). The fragment optimization stage involves building fragment hits into novel ligands (*de novo* drug design), prediction of binding pose (molecular docking, molecular dynamics), and prediction of binding affinity (scoring functions). Further stages for candidate leads can include structure-based drug design (docking, scoring and molecular dynamics) and ligand-based drug design (pharmacophore, QSAR and focused libraries).

It is possible to do good work using fragment docking combined with expanded sampling. Fragment-specific scoring functions may be necessary however to improve binding energy predictions. Fragments have less hydrogen bond donors and acceptors, less rotable bonds, more translational and rotational freedom. Thus, care should be taken to calculate entropic contributions [151]. The concept of 'ligandability' (where high values indicates that a protein is likely to bind fragments with good affinity) can be used to estimate binding to targets by docking fragments.

It is possible to evaluate each fragment of a decomposed compound *via* a pre-docked database. Each fragment ranked according to specific interactions with the receptor. New compounds can be formed replacing and reassembling the best binding fragments to yield improved analogs. If a sufficient number of fragments are used, fragment docking should give good results [150-229].

CONSENSUS DOCKING

There are a number of well-established and successful strategies in the literature for discovering protein ligands. The strategies are twofold. First, the compounds screened/docked into the active site of a protein structure model yields conformation, location and orientation (pose). Subsequently, the pose is used to calculate a predicted binding affinity of the compound with the protein. The accuracy of the score is dependent on the accuracy of the predicted binding pose. The virtual screening method has the limitation that significantly different poses can yield similar docking scores (without possibility of distinguishing the correct pose). The hit rates of virtual screening obtained from incorrect poses results in incorrect affinity predictions.

Predicting affinity of a compound for a protein is challenging. In order to reduce the error it is common to combine the results of several scoring algorithms into a consensus-scoring scheme. Consequently, we have consensus scoring which is a method whereas binding affinities of compounds for a particular target are predicted using more than one scoring algorithm. This could be superior in accuracy as compared to the usage of single algorithms [230, 231].

This can proceed from the fact that structure-based *in silico* prediction of ligand binding affinity involves two steps. It starts with prediction of the ligand pose (correct pose should match the pose in a crystallized protein or enzyme). Subsequently, binding affinities close to experimental observations predicted. Correct binding conformation should be used as input if scoring algorithms are to predict the affinity of a ligand correctly.

A greater increase in accuracy can be obtained when combining dissimilar types of scoring functions in contrast to combining similar types. The combination of an empirical with a knowledge-based scoring method compensates for the other's weaknesses. Programs calibrated using different training data sets are complementary since they are able to draw on a larger body of statistical information.

The dual approach could be applied to virtual screening methods, for example, by docking the compound library first with one method and then with another. Subsequently, the predicted binding poses compared with the criteria that those that agree should have a higher chance of being correct and passed on to the following drug discovery stage.

BIOISOSTERIC REPLACEMENTS

Bioisosterism suggests two bioisosteric compounds have a shape that is similar in terms of a particular biological environment, *i.e.* a protein-binding site [232-243]. They are substructures or molecules with the same number of valence electrons and atoms, similar physiochemical properties, near-equal molecular shapes and volumes, approximately the same distribution of electrons. Biososteric compounds affect the same biochemically associated systems and thereby produce biological properties related to each other.

The variation of the functional groups within a candidate ligand is one of the approaches in drug design to improve multiple molecular properties. It provides an indication of the characteristics of different substituent replacements, allowing the determination of areas where no further exploration may be necessary.

Bioisosterism makes it possible for us to make informed modifications to potential new drug compounds in order to alter key properties such as solubility or toxicity while the activity of a molecule is improved or maintained. This increases the chances of success and culmination in a viable drug candidate.

Despite developments of specialized computational tools, appropriate bioisosteric modification is a challenging task that still relies to some extent on the experience and intuition of the chemist. The chemical physical properties required in a modification to maintain a molecule's potency depends on which properties of the original fragment contributed to this activity. The toxicity and solubility can also alter as a function of the scaffold where attached.

Similar fragments, in their chemical-physical properties, should act as more robust bioisosteric replacements in contrast with strongly differing fragments. Methods have evolved to detect interchangeable pairs based on data analysis and similarity. Larger weights are assigning to replacements that incorporate information about the system. These features could be present in replacements and less importance assigned to other features. We note that similarity is not limited to well-known replacements. It is also necessary to focus on the similarity in the portion of property-space that underlies the compound's activity [232-243].

Approaches such as principal component analysis, self-organizing maps and nonlinear mapping are methods used to discover a lower-dimensional embedding of a high-dimensional space. It offers the medicinal chemist an easier visualization of the entire space considered. 'Hammett's σ' constant and 'Hansch's π parameter' play important roles in characterization of functional groups since they characterize/explain the electron-donating power and hydrophobicity of the considered substituents. Once attention is paid to the points of attachment, it is possible to calculate thousands of molecular descriptors of response. Many of these descriptors were already developed for early QSAR research [232, 233].

Various approaches can also describe steric properties of substituents. The simplest is to count the number of atoms or the molecular weight of the substituent as well as summing the van der Waals radii of the substituents atoms and even taking into account the distance between attachment points. A simple approach to predict the hydrogen-bonding potential of a substituent is to simple encode the number of hydrogen bond acceptors (HBA) and hydrogen bond donors (HBD).

Often the molecular field of a substituent is characterized as descriptors encoding pharmacophoric feature points and their relations, orientations or electrostatic potentials. When possible, conformational flexibility is taking into consideration. Another interesting approach is the mining of bioisosteric groups from molecular databases with biological activities yielding a rich resource of chemically feasible bioisosteric pairs. This yields novel relative orientations and combinations of substituents permitting even local exploration of the chemical space of interest.

There are procedures for automated extraction of transformation rules for bioisosteric replacements. The determination of a pair of substituents that are bioisosterically equivalent is still a challenging area of research. Another area of interest is the identification of bioisosteric groups based on similarity of group properties. The challenge of scaffold hopping is a subset of bioisosteric replacement [232-243].

SCAFFOLD HOPPING

The aim of scaffold hoping is to discover structural novel compounds starting from known active compounds by modifying the central core structure of the molecule. The term scaffold describe the core structure of a molecule. The core structure is the central component of a molecule, the substantial substructure that contains the molecular material necessary to ensure that the functional groups are in a desired geometrical arrangement [244-254].

Hit selection and lead generation are major research areas of medicinal chemistry. Ligand complexity, ligand-binding efficiency, chemical tractability and ligand-target profile are important parameters in hit selection. More chemistry resources could be devoted to scaffold modifications to expand the candidate pool in lead generation.

Since many druggable targets are promiscuous towards lipophilic ligands, it may be interesting to modify the hydrophobic portions of hit compounds in scaffold and analog design. Scaffold hopping is also defined as a computational technique that identifies compounds containing a topogically different scaffold from the parent compound with, however, improved or similar activity from a given database. Very simple or complex compounds may require drastic changes, *i.e.* more scaffolds may be required to validate, synthesize or invalidate chemistry-demanding efforts.

There is still a limited number of druggable targets. Their exploration is based on known ligands or protein-ligand structures. Based on this knowledge, the question then is how to design economically viable drugs maintaining or improving efficiency and pharmacokinetic (PK) profiles of existing therapies by designing novel structural scaffolds.

Effectively, one of the strategies for discovering structurally novel compounds is lead hopping (scaffold hopping), a relatively young concept applied from the beginning of drug discovery. The method starts with known active compounds yielding novel chemotypes by modifying the central core structure of the molecules. Often modification of side chains is sufficient to overcome undesirable properties associated with parent molecules. On the contrary it may be necessary to modify the core structure of the scaffold.

The concept of scaffold hopping was introduced as a technique to identify isofunctional molecular structures with significant different molecular backbones emphasizing two key components. These are core structures and similar biological activities of the new compounds relative to the parent compounds. Scaffold hopping can also be classified into four groups, *i.e.* heterocycle replacements, topology-based hopping, peptidomimetics and ring opening or closure.

Derivatives obtained from the parent compounds having novel core structures can define scaffold hopping. However, how different should the derivative molecules be from the parent in order to classify as scaffold hopping the resultant evolution? For this purpose, we can focus on the degree of change associated with the original parent molecule, whereas minor modifications such as replacing or swapping carbon and heteroatoms in a backbone ring is classified as a first hop. More extensive ring opening and closures are classified as a second hop. Replacements of peptide backbones with nonpeptic moieties falls into the category of a third hop. Complete new chemical backbones that only retain interactions are characterized as a fourth hop.

In the heterocycle replacement or first hop, we have heterocycles functioning as cores of drug molecules usually providing multiple vectors projecting to different directions. Replacing the C-carbon, N-nitrogen, O = oxygen and S = sulfur atoms in a heterocycle while maintaining the outreaching vectors can result in novel scaffolds. This yields improved binding affinity when there is involvement of the heterocycles with the target protein.

Pseudo ring structures constitute the second hop. Since most drug-like molecules contain at least one ring system, ring closure and opening are immediate strategies to create novel scaffolds with drug-like properties. The molecular flexibility contributes considerable to entropic components of the binding free energy as well as to membrane penetration and absorption. By controlling the total number of free rotatable bonds, ring opening and closure it is possible to manipulate the flexibility of a molecule.

Pseudopeptides and peptidomimetics constitute the third hop. Peptides that are biologically active such as hormones, neuropeptides and growth factors have important biological functions in our bodies. Unbalance can yield diabetes, osteoporosis and cancer. The major goal of peptide-based drug discovery is to reduce the peptide character to enhance the resistance to proteolysis, while maintaining the key chemical features for molecular recognition. A typical method used to perform the peptide to small molecule transition is scaffold hopping.

Topology/shape-based scaffold hopping defines the fourth hop. This is often generated using a virtual screening. Ultimately, scaffold hopping focuses on discovering novel core structures often ignoring potential conflicts between side chains and targets.

Scaffold hopping can be a useful tool for overcoming undesirable properties such as toxicity and poor exposure. Future software developments in scaffold hoping is needed to incorporate guiding elements for achieving acceptable pharmacological properties such as better PK profiles, reduced toxicity and improved absorption. This could enable a generalized scaffold-hopping approach, which maximizes the chemical diversity maintaining or even improving the biological activity and pharmacological profiles of the original drug [244-254].

PHARMACOPHORE MODELING

Pharmacophore modeling is a very useful medicinal chemistry tool for the design of therapeutic agents (new chemical entities). The concept was first introduced in the beginning of the last century. It was defined as a molecular framework that carries 'phoros'. These are the essential features responsible for a drug's biological activity (phorons). These concepts have evolved/matured to a better comprehension of the properties of ligand structures/targets.

The modern concept defines pharmacophores as an ensemble of steric and electronic features necessary to ensure optimal interactions with specific biological structures and trigger/block their biological response [255]. They can be important in the search for molecules on targets. When used as *in silico* filters, they can reduce substantially the cost and number of compounds processed in subsequent stages. One does this by focusing on local similarity, studying the specific arrangements and molecular determinants necessary for biological activity processes and providing explanations for the predicted activity of molecules. In order words, pharmacophores reflects how medicinal chemists can characterize the binding ability of molecular ligands to biological targets.

The initial application of the pharmacophore hypothesis were two dimensional. Tools were used in order to identify privileged motifs associated with biological activity; explore/understand structure-activity relationships and guide the synthesis of new bioactive compounds. However, these pharmacophores, with strict constraints and restrictions, retrieved only highly related structural analogues. Advances with these protocols have been obtained with the development of three dimensional (3D) pharmacophores. The concept is based on the interactions that define the binding of a ligand to a receptor. Charge transfer, hydrogen bonding, hydrophobic and electrostatic interactions can be grouped and aligned in 3D space. A common arrangement of stereo-electronic features can be generated which are essential for ligand binding to a target defining the key interactions responsible for molecular recognition/affinity/biological activity.

The three-dimensional pharmacophores have diversified applications in drug discovery. These applications include aligning molecules using modeling algorithms; retrieving molecules with similar stereo-electronic properties from databases; guiding the virtual docking of compounds and building *de novo* virtual compound libraries. Issues such as ADME/Tox properties can also be addressed.

Currently it is possible to design drugs from the information obtained from both ligands and targets. There are consequently, two fundamental approaches or pharmacophore perception, *i.e.* ligand-based and structure-based pharmacophores [255-269]. Contributing strongly to the drug discovery and design process, LBPs (ligand-based pharmacophores) are derived from multiple active ligands. Bioactive compounds can be used as templates to derive hypothesis for the search of new scaffolds with similar or enhanced biological activity.

On the other hand, increasing attention is also given to SBPs (structure-based pharmacophores). These are obtained from 3d structures of protein targets as a result of the increase in high resolution protein structures (Protein Data-bank). Based on the conformation and arrangement of the receptor, pharmacophore models can be generated. These can take into account both the physicochemical features and the space complementarity of the ligand-receptor binding site. Pharmacophore decriptors derived from receptor binding sites enables common reference frames for both ligand and receptors. Complementary pharmacophore features to the binding sites defines images that represents the ideal ligands. Models and fingerpints can be derived and used to discover new biological active compounds. The spatial arrangement of the amino acids within the binding site specify physicochemical and structural constraints that should be met by any putative ligand. The traditional 'lock and key' paradigm can provide satisfactory results for biologically active rigid sites or conformation-selective inhibitors.

SBP's can be used for target fishing (find new targets for specific ligands). They can yield insight into ligand-protein interactions, ligand-protein interactions and enable ligand profiling (structural chemogenomics studies aimed at identification of new ligands for specific proteins). They can allow identification of novel scaffolds, elucidation of protein-ligand chemotypes/binding modes, provide tools for structure-based ligand optimization and increase comprehension of binding sites. They can also find ligands for orphan receptors and allow cross-pharmacology applications in order to suggest new targets for existing drugs.

We can divide the preparation of SBPs into four major steps, *i.e.* protein structure preparation, binding site detection; pharmacophore feature definition and selection. At the protein, backbone, polar hydrogen atoms, side chains potential conformation, and protonation states variations are expected to be larger making the selection of pharmacophore features more complex than in ligand-based pharmacophores.

The pre-requisite for SBP method is the availability of a 3d protein structure. Subsequently, protein structure preparation is required (including non-protein groups such as water molecules, determination of protonation states, position of hydrogen atoms and consideration of protein conformations). The biologically active ligand conformation is typically used to align multiple active molecules and deduce a pharmacophore. Subsequently it is necessary to define the location of the ligand-binding site using appropriate algorithms. In a subsequent stage, pharmacophore features can be obtained from co-crystallized ligands or ligand binding sites.

Favorable interactions can be characterized by geometric entities, spheres, vectors and planes and common interaction types include H-bond acceptors, H-bond donors, ionizable groups, aromatic rings and liphophilic regions. For compound library enrichment and binding mode hypothesis, it is necessary to select features, which correlate with biological activity. Protein-ligand interaction energies can estimate and prioritize interactions and discard those with small contributions to the overall binding energy. Probe docking can select features at positions where probes have high interaction energies. If multiple ligands are available and binding mode hypothesis generated, features, which correlate with conserved protein-ligand interactions can be identified.

Selection of important binding site amino acid residues can be done through evaluation of sequence variations. Known active compounds can be used to select specific combinations of pharmacophore features and include shape restraints in the SBP model. Shape and volume restraints are important concepts for virtual screening and lead optimizations. SBPs can be used to improve molecular understanding of ligand-protein interactions, virtual screening, ligand binding mode prediction and binding site similarity detection. Ligand- and protein structure-based methods are complementary approaches for identifying different ligand chemotypes suggesting models that are a combination of LBP and SBPs. X-ray crystallizations and NMR spectroscopy are well suited for combination with SBPs.

SBPs can be detected by a number of methods. These include grid generation, molecular dynamics, protein-ligand complexes, overlay based clustering, homology models, chemoprints and geometry-based models. They can also help understand the interaction of ligands with proteins, affinity/selectivity prediction, hit optimization, structure-activity relationships, binding pocket exploration, targeting excluded residues, correct ligand binding prediction and even compare ligand-binding sites.

Geometric methods to derive SBPs are often the least restrictive. This protocol together with the probe-based method are the approaches applied in the absence of known ligands. Reduction of the high number of features is a challenge in SBP in order to obtain characteristic of biological activity interest. Energy based methods depend on the accuracy of input/binding modes. Statistical protocols can work with low quality structures. The pharmacophore concept is relatively simple yielding an attractive tool for research applications [255-269]. Discovery Studio (Accelrys software) is one of the softwares for pharmacophe modeling. In the sections on docking and virtual screening programs we describe fitty one programs that use diversified protocols including pharmacophores.

INDUCED FIT

Different mechanisms can play a role in the variety of conformational changes occurring upon protein-ligand binding. The term induced fit is used to describe the resultant tight structural complementarity of the interaction partners taken into consideration by docking methods. Handling the protein as flexible is not common and still remains a challenge in contrast to ligand flexibility in docking protocols. This is particularly true, if we consider computational difficulties/time involved [270-319].

Important for protein function and ligand binding is protein flexibility. At finite temperatures, this can result in numerous motions including rotations about single bonds up to large-scale collective movements of loops, secondary structure elements or even entire domains. Binding can depend on motion in certain parts of the protein, affect flexibility of the protein (altering its dynamics properties), modulating the possibilities of motion and compensate as well for unfavorable entropic contributions from molecular interactions.

The ability of binding partners to have conformational adaption to each other, *i.e.* plasticity, is important for docking whereas ligands can adopt a conformation suitable for tight interaction with their target protein that often does not correspond to the lowest energy conformation of the ligand. Proteins can also have a variety of changes on binding from small side chain adaptations to large domain movements.

The concept of induced fit is often used to describe any conformational change in a protein due to ligand binding whereas the well-known lock-and-key principle should remain valid (mutual adaptation).

The model of conformational selection challenges induced fit whereas the protein conformational ensemble is re-distributed upon binding giving preference to population of states resulting in a net gain in free energy. However, even if conformational selection is the actual mechanism, the ligand induces the observable conformational changes.

Since protein and ligand are generally not in the adopted complex conformation, a central problem is the conformational flexibility of both proteins and ligands. Fragment-based and whole-molecule approaches are two general strategies used to handle ligand flexibility. The latter addressed as an extension of rigid-docking (separate docking of pre-calculated ligand conformations). Due to the large increase of possible conformers, the latter method may be less suited for molecules that are flexible.

Subjecting the initial matches to an optimization/conformational relaxation is another way of accounting partially for conformational flexibility. Another method consists of sampling ligand conformation space during docking with the corresponding disadvantage of high computational demands. Usage of internal coordinates could also help reduce the number of variables involved.

Another general method is fragment-based whereas the molecule is divided into fragments to be rigidly docked individually and then reconnected or built-up incrementally. The method uses incremental construction algorithms, *i.e.* anchor and grow which has the advantage of potential elimination of combinations at an early stage.

Due to computational demands, incorporation of protein flexibility is still challenging in docking and virtual screening calculations where there is a large number of degrees of freedom to be considered. More sophisticated algorithms and heuristics are required, incorporating for example, previous knowledge of the system.

We can use different criteria for handling protein flexibility. Considering the degree of flexibility there could be a distinction between side-chain flexibility, global flexibility and loop flexibility. It could also be more closely related to the methodology, *i.e.* implicit consideration of plasticity, modeling of side-chain conformational changes in the binding pocket and large scale conformational changes including backbend motions.

Focusing on methodological aspects, a detailed classification into five categories can be made. These categories are soft methods to reduce penalties from steric clashes; methods based on the selection of a small set of essential degrees of freedom in the binding site; ensemble-based methods; molecular simulation methods modified for flexible receptor docking and methods based on collective degrees of freedom.

Full induced-fit docking approaches for moderate plasticity are becoming available yielding non-prohibitive docking applications including side-chain modeling and automated approaches. However if complicated energetic effects are involved, small conformational changes of few side chains may yield unexpected results. More progress is also required for scoring (localized backbone motions as well as flexible-protein docking benchmarking) [270-320].

CHEMOGENOMIC APPROACHES

Only a very small fraction of compounds describing the current chemical space has been tested on an also very small fraction of the entire target space. Chemogenomics is an interdisciplinary field. It attempts to match target and ligand space and ultimately identify ligands of targets. Receptors are grouped into sets of related receptor families that can be explored in a systematic manner and derive predictive links between the chemical structures of receptors and interacting bioactive molecules.

Regarding chemogenomics, we note that there are various definitions of overlapping fields (chemical genetics, chemical genomics). A broad definition of chemogenomics encompasses chemoproteomics (the study of small-molecular-weight drug candidates on gene/protein function). Chemogenomics is at the interface of chemistry, biology and informatics (data mining). Borderline methodologies (medicinal chemistry, chemoinformatics, bioinformatics) play major roles in bringing these major disciplines together.

For drug discovery, chemogenomic approaches to drug discovery require target/compound libraries, high-throughput binding and functional assays or gene/protein expressions.

Predictive chemogenomics can attempt to predict compounds-genes/proteins relationships, target selectivity for various ligands as well as ligand selectivity for various targets. It can span pure ligand-based approaches (comparison of known ligands to predict their most probable targets), pure target-based approaches (comparison of targets or ligand-binding sites to predict their most likely ligands) or ultimately target-ligand based approaches to predict binding affinities.

Effectively, chemogenomic techniques can be used to profile small molecules against large collections of macromolecular structures in order to identify proteins. These can in turn bind to the referred molecules (target fishing). Chemogenomics approaches can also determine a global pharmacological profile (ligand profiling) as complementary ways to increase the productivity of drug discovery. Typical approaches are poised towards identification of new ligands for a target. For inverse virtual screening, each single ligand is compared against a collection of targets. This can yield fruitful drug discovery rewards for ligand profiling and target fishing [321, 322].

Chemogenomics approaches can also help to identify new molecular targets for compounds (in clinical trials or for existing drugs called drug repositioning aggregating more volumes of polypharmacological data). It is of interest to develop semantic web technologies in order to link different diseases. Chemogenomic approaches can also be used for modeling and predicting pharmacokinetics features of compounds, which can be profiled for focused testing and screening of the promising compounds. This would reduce risks of late-stage attrition and reduce overall costs.

The chemogenomics approach can provide tools that permit the prediction of toxicity and crucial ADME-Tox properties including volume of distribution, clearance, metabolism, plasma protein binding and transporters [321-323].

KNOWLEDGE-BASED DRUG DISCOVERY

Biopharmaceutical companies need more ways to screen for potential problems with promising molecules at the earliest possible stage. It is important to streamline the entire process such that compounds move quickly along the development pipeline. There is great need for more solutions that can transform data into knowledge.

Automated techniques are necessary to manage and analyze the huge amount of data in chemical/biological databases. KBDD (Knowledge-based drug discovery) can be used to extract from databases useful and novel knowledge units. The core of the KBDD process is data mining that involves applying algorithms to explore data and discover significant patterns yielding 'knowledge units' [324-338].

Effectively, knowledge discovery (data mining), is a computer-assisted process which consists of digging through/analyzing huge sets of data. Subsequently, the 'meaning' of the data is extracted. Effectively, these tools can predict behaviors as well as future trends. This can help scientists to make knowledge-driven decisions. Data mining tools can yield many answers that are too time consuming traditionally. They go through databases for hidden patterns. It is possible to find predictive information (outside expectations) that experts may miss. The name has its origin from the similarities between searching a large database for valuable information and mining for a valuable ore in a mountain. Both processes require sifting or intelligently probing through considerable material to find answers.

KBDD, for example, can enhance 3DVS by applying machine-learning techniques to 3D information regarding ligands, proteins and their corresponding interactions. Nonetheless, the KBDD process needs training on a data set (active and inactive compounds). The automation of this training set is not evident. KBDD can be used with protein-ligand interactions for the following purposes: a) design scoring functions, b) target focused libraries, c) target databases of known active ligands to derive physicochemical, structural and ADME-Tox property profiles [324-338].

As an example, absorption, distribution, metabolism, excretion, and toxicity data is important for developing reliable *in silico* ADMET models. Contributing to this effort a pharmacokinetics knowledge base (PKKB) database was reported which compile comprehensive information about ADMET properties into a single electronic repository. This database contains more than 10 000 experimental ADMET measurements of 1685 drugs, including octanol/water partition coefficient, solubility, dissociation constant, intestinal absorption, Caco-2 permeability, human bioavailability, plasma protein binding, blood-plasma partitioning ratio, volume of distribution, metabolism, half-life, excretion, urinary excretion, clearance, toxicity, half lethal dose in rat or mouse, *etc* [40].

For new target families, chemical knowledge has to be generated. Beyond biological target validation, the emphasis is on chemistry/physics to provide the molecules (for which novel biology/pharmacology can be studied).

BINDING AFFINITY PREDICTION

The affinity of the ligand compound to the macromolecular receptor is assumed closely related to its biological activity. Consequently, the key for computational lead optimization is the accurate prediction of the ligand-receptor binding affinities.

The essential components for determining affinity include contributions from solvation and desolvation, electrostatic interactions between the ligand and the receptor; enthalpic and entropic contributions resulting from changes in the number of degrees of freedom; conformational changes of ligand and receptor experienced upon complex formation and spatial complementarity of both binding partners.

In the absence of consonance regarding reliability/efficiency of methods to predict affinities, whereas the most accurate are also more time-consuming, many approaches are used for adapting different requirements to evaluate affinities [324,339-361]. More details will be discussed in the following sections.

Scoring Functions

Computational tools such as docking play an important role in drug design whereas an important problem is the determination and development of energy scoring functions that can describe accurately the ligand-protein interactions [107, 142, 148, 295, 303, 304, 327, 331, 332, 346, 355, 358, 362-554].

There are typically three applications of the energy scoring functions in molecular docking.

   a)   Determination of the ligand site and its binding mode for a protein. By
         evaluating the strength of the binding, molecular docking generates

for a protein target many putative binding conformations/orientations at the protein's active site. A scoring function is then used to rank the ligand orientations. The experimental binding mode would be of course more highly ranked by an ideal scoring function.

b) Prediction of absolute binding affinity between ligand and protein. In lead optimization, the strength of binding affinities for selected compounds (lead compounds or low-affinity hits) is improved.

c) For a given protein target, identification of potential drug/leads *via* screening of databases. Known binders are ranked highly by reliable scoring functions. Virtual database screening, binding affinity prediction and ligand binding mode identification are interconnected such that equal performance for all three applications are obtained by an accurate scoring function.

We can also group the scoring functions in a) force field-based, b) empirical, c) knowledge-based.

a) The first type, *i.e.* FF (force field scoring functions) are based on physical chemical like atomic interactions. These include electrostatic, van der Waals (VDW) interactions as well as torsional/bond stretching/bending forces. The functions and their parameters can be obtained from *ab initio* quantum mechanical calculations or/and experimental data. The solvent is a challenging problem. The Lennard-Jones VDW and the electrostatic terms of the force field energy components ($1/\epsilon r_{ij}^2$ as well as (r_{ij}^{-6}), (r_{ij}^{-12}) pairwise distance dependent terms respectively.

The effect of the solvent is implicitly introduced by a dielectric constant, which is dependent on distance. This dielectric factor cannot account for desolvation effects because non-polar groups tend to remain in non-aqueous environment and charged groups favor aqueous environments. Desolvation energy depends on specific geometric and chemical environments of solute atoms. It is a many body problem. Scoring functions would be biased on Coulomb electrostatic interactions (tend to select highly charged ligands) if we ignore desolvation effects.

Consequently, it is more accurate to explicitly treat water molecules. This can be done with computationally expensive free energy and thermodynamic integration methods. We must keep in mind however that the overall accuracy of the method is still limited by accuracy of force fields as well as sampling protocols. Here the mathematical form of the parameterization is very important. Improved force field models can be introduced using a continuum dielectric medium. Poisson-Boltzmann/surface area model (PB/SA) and the generalized-Born surface area (GB/SA) are examples of these models which can be used for post-scoring. These will be discussed again in following chapters.

It is also necessary to understand how to combine individual energy terms. Empirical weighting coefficients are often used since the Lennard-Jones potentials, the electrostatic components and hydrophobic interactions terms are on different scales. Experimental data is is fitted to yield weighting factors. It is however difficult to determine universal sets of weights for ligand-protein complexes. It is also necessary to consider poor treatment of entropic contribution and the fact that the free energy terms may not be additive.

b) Empirical scoring functions estimate the binding affinity by summation over sets of weighed energy terms such as electrostatics, VDW energies, desolvation, hydrogen bonds, hydrophobicity, entropy, *etc*. Calculation of the scoring functions is relatively fast. Empirical scoring function also include diverse terms. These are as follows: ionic interactions; lipophilic protein-ligand contact surface; number of rotable bonds in the ligand; number and geometry of intermolecular hydrogen bonds; ionic interaction; flexibility of the ligand; electrostatic potential in the binding site; water molecules in the binding site; cavities along the protein-ligand interface; specific interactions between aromatic rings; metal atoms and effective number of rotatable bonds in the ligand.

Many protein-ligand programs use different empirical energy terms in their empirical scoring functions. Training sets may be necessary to avoid problems such as double counting.

c)   Knowledge-based scoring functions are also known as statistical-potential based scoring functions. Here energy potentials (can be derived with experimental information) are used. Using the inverse Boltzmann relation, pairwise potentials can be directly obtained from the occurrence frequency of atom pairs. In the simple fluid system, by the inverse Boltzmann method, the interaction potentials are the mean-force potentials. For complex protein systems, the Boltzmann method can convert a histogram of atom-atom distances into a suitable function with the dimensions of energy.

The knowledge-based scoring function potentials are extracted from structures to reproduce the known affinities by fitting. They are robust and quite insensitive to training sets. In addition, the scoring process can be as fast as using empirical scoring functions. The disadvantage is the challenge of reference states. Often the reference state is approximated by an atom-randomized state by ignoring effects such as excluded volume and interatomic connectivity. Some scoring functions consists of a distance-dependent pair-potential term and a surface-dependent single potential term. Corrections or scaling can also be introduced to improve the accuracy of the reference states. The potential of mean force (PMF) is one of the first knowledge-based scoring functions extensively tested for affinity [547].

The problem of the reference state is a problem using either more physical approximations or atom-randomized states. The pairwise potentials are not sensitive enough to ligand positions highlighting the problem for virtual screening and binding mode predictions. Consequently, a knowledge-based potential scoring function was developed (ITScore) in which the requirement of accurate reference state calculations is avoided [548]. The pair potential can be iteratively adjusted to reproduce experimental training set distribution functions, which are able to discriminate decoys from native structures. A set of well-sampled decoys as well as an ensemble of the native structures is used to predict the pair distribution function. The full binding energy landscapes of the complexes are thus included. Solvation and configuration entropy effects can also be included.

Another method is the consensus scoring [230, 231]. Taking into account general applicability and accuracy, none of the protocols are 'ideal/perfect'. With the objective of increasing the probability of finding better lead compounds/correct solutions, consensus-scoring protocols were introduced. These models attempt to balance the deficiencies of some techniques and use the advantages of other procedures. However, in order to discrimination lead compounds/binders and true modes, it is necessary to design appropriate consensus scoring strategies of the individual scores. Typical strategies include number-by-number, vote-by number, linear combination, average rank, *etc*.

It is necessary to adopt good criteria to evaluate the ability of a scoring function to predict binding affinity, identify modes and do successful virtual database screening. It is important for scoring functions to be able to distinguish decoys from native binding giving the highest ranking to the native structures. The rmsd values between experiment (native structure) and predictions of native binding are typically used to evaluate successful docking applications. This model is relatively simple and easy to implement. However, random placements, nearly symmetrical or small ligands activities can yield equally good values. In addition, the rmsd protocol may not yield good binding mode predictions for solvent exposed large flexible ligands.

For pose evaluations, alternative protocols were introduced to overcome limitations. These methods include real space R-factor (RSR), generally applicable replacement for rmsd (GARD), relative displacement error (RDE) and interaction based accuracy classification (IBAC) [342, 548-550].

It is also important for the scoring function to measure the strength of the binding between the ligand and the protein. It may not be very feasible to scale scores to experimental binding data. It may be more feasible to scale them to fit the normal affinity range. The Pearson correlation is commonly used for evaluation of affinity prediction scoring of experimental data. This correlation method is an arithmetic average over all the complexes taking into consideration the number of tested complexes (N), the experimentally determined binding energies as well as the calculated scores for all the complexes.

The prediction of binding affinity is more challenging due in part to the origin of the experimental values (different experimental conditions, research groups, inherent experimental errors).

It is also possible to evaluate scoring from the capability of selecting and accurately ranking hits from databases. The accumulated rate of active hits found above a percentage of the ranked database (binders and inactive ligands) yields the enrichment. Maintaining a fixed percentage, a higher enrichment indicates a better scoring function.

Using AUC is another procedure for evaluation scoring in virtual database screening, *i.e.* using the area under the receiver operating characteristic curve (ROC) [551]. In cases when the number of active binders is comparable to the inactive ligands, this method could be more appropriate. Due to inherent limitations, most scoring functions should, but do not perform well for all the procedures previously discussed. It is noteworthy that good binding affinity prediction is not equivalent to good database ranking.

Construction of appropriate test/training sets is also important for evaluating scoring. High quality/resolution structures are prioritized. Whenever possible diverse protein type and a wide range of binding affinities should be used. Bond-covalent binding and drug-like ligands should be prioritized. It is important to avoid training/test sets overlaps. Publicly available benchmarks (CSAR/, (http://csardock.org), DUD (http://dud.docking.org) and others are invaluable.

In 2013 it was reported a comparison of neural-network scoring functions and the state of the art applications to common library screening. Neural networks are computer models expected to mimic the microscopic architecture and organization of the brain. There is *in silico* simulation of biological neurons and connections. Data encoded on the neurodes and signals are propagated through the network. The number of neurodes and weights are used to modify the initial input signal propagation. In the output layer of artificial neurons, analysis of the original input signal is ultimately encoded [346]. For scoring evaluations the strengths of the connection between neurodes can be varied until the network could reliably predict binding affinities when given descriptors of ligand-receptor complexes.

A specific receptor tailored composite scoring function has been designed to optimize ranking of known inhibitors can potentially enhance virtual-screening performance. The best protocol to use in a virtual-screening project is highly dependent on the target receptor studied.

Recent work suggest improving the scoring of protein-ligand binding affinity by including the effects of structural water and electronic polarization. The authors use minimization, MD, MM/PBSA and their incorporated specific charge model (PPC) to obtain correct ranking of binding poses in which bridging water molecules and electronic polarization play an important role [553].

Recent studies report optimization of molecular docking scores with 'support vector rank regression' (SVM), a statistical learning strategy that in principle represents a major advance in machine leaning methodology [554]. SVM uses training examples to construct a decision hyperplane in a high-dimensional feature space. The decision margin is maximized in order to minimize the generalization error. It is often implemented as a classification algorithm that learns from categorical examples to classify new instances.

It is also implemented as a regression algorithm that learns from continuously varying examples to predict the target value of new instances. Using different example datasets and training strategies the authors conclude that with additional features for comparative fitness between computed binding conformations, the algorithm holds the potential to create a new category of more accurate integrative docking scores.

ENTROPIC CONTRIBUTIONS

A long-standing challenge is the rigorous evaluation of entropic fluctuations during macromolecular associations in molecular modeling. Effectively, ligand

and receptor flexibility and corresponding entropic contributions to binding free energies are important in docking/scoring stages. Since accurate force fields as well as specialized/extensive sampling procedures are required, rigorous free energy simulation are far from trivial, requiring expertise and computational power. Since entropy is physically rooted in statistical thermodynamics, sampling requirements are crucial. Entropic effects are intimately related with protein flexibility particularly if ligand binding results in changes of the number of available torsional degrees of freedom [339-364].

Free energy calculations, at a computational cost, may be useful for assigning weights to individual receptor conformations as well as better/improved free energy estimates. Hardware/software computational progress, ongoing methodological developments, new algorithms and systematic validation against calorimetric experimental data could eventually yield more routine usage of free energy calculations. These topics will be discussed in more detail in the following sections.

MOLECULAR DYNAMICS

In order to predict the interactions of elastic hard spheres models, Alder and Wainwright performed in the late 1950's one of the first molecular dynamics (MD) simulations [555-576]. In 1959 Gibson *et al.* performed the MD of a real material (radiation damage in Cu) [556]. Rahman (dynamics of liquid argon) did one of the first simulations by MD of a real system in liquid in 1964 [557]. Development in the 1970's, MD simulations were done in more complex systems (bovine pancreatic trypsin inhibitor) by McCammon. With the increase of computing power, MD is used in numerous fields of science by different groups all over the world with an increasing number of publications regarding applications and theory.

MD, a conformation search procedure, is one of the principal tools in theoretical studies of biological molecules. It is a conformation space search. In this procedure, the atoms of the biological macromolecule gets an initial velocity and then allowed, according to Newtonian mechanics, to evolve in time. Depending on the simulated temperature, the macromolecule can subsequently, overcome barriers found in the surface of potential energy. The picture of the dynamics molecular conformations can be provided by this procedure.

A static picture can be provided by using a procedure based on simple energy minimization. A complete description of molecular motions on the sub-picosecond time scales is obtained by this procedure providing important information for the system investigated. This information may be only partially accessible through experimental techniques. A knowledge of the molecule's dynamics can yield a complete understanding of the structure-function relationship.

It is advisable to do an energy minimization before starting a MD simulation. This allows the energy to equilibrate among the constituent atoms, remove van der Waals interaction, avoid/reduce local structural distortion and unstable stimulations, kinetic energies and thermal noise in the structures and potential energies.

These minimization methods are classified as first derivative whereas only the first derivative of the potential energy function is calculated. In the second-derivate methods, both the first and second derivatives are calculated as done in the Newton-Raphson method [558]. The steepest descent is a simple method of minimization. The conjugate gradient method minimizes the function of energy potential in successive steps in order to achieve the minimum point whereas information is saved to guide subsequent steps. Hessian matrix techniques are used in the Newton-Ralphson methods with a high computational cost.

When we do molecular dynamics simulations, there is a computation of the molecular potential energy taken as a sum of energy terms. There is a description of the deviation (away from equilibrium values) of torsion angles, bond lengths and bond angles. Electrostatic and van der Waals interactions are also described by other terms. It is important to carefully determine the equilibrium bond angles, partial charge, bond lengths, Van der Waals parameters and force constants. This is obtained by fitting to high-level quantum mechanical calculations or experimental data. Combination of methods for free energy predictions with MD simulations yields a good strategy for identifying interactions for drug design.

There are various levels of theory to study structures and properties of bio molecular systems. The systems can be described in quantum mechanical methods by wave functions of the Schrodinger equation, which relates the Hamiltonian operator to the stationary states, and energies of the system. However, approximations should be made since the Schrodinger equation cannot be solved exactly in practice.

With the exception of using fundamental constants of nature, *i.e.* Planck's constants and the mass of the electron, approximations of the solution of the Schrodinger equation are called *ab initio*. It is possible to use these methods to determine quite accurately electrostatic potential and molecular structures. However, the applications of these methods are limited to small systems due to heavy computational demands.

Biomolecular systems have too many electronic degrees of freedom for solving the Schrodinger's equation. The sophisticated molecular modeling techniques are too computational demanding when large systems comprising hundreds/thousands of atoms are involved, in contrast to molecular dynamics simulations.

MD is a method based on molecular mechanics, which calculates the molecular system's behavior in a time dependent procedure. It is considered as a virtual experiment or an interface between theory and laboratory experiment. These methods can be used to get a better understanding of biophysical and biochemical processes. They also yield a better comprehension of factors determining structural stability by sampling efficiently the configuration space. These methods are useful for understanding small molecules (drugs), biomolecular structures as well as their interactions.

In molecular mechanical methods it is assumed that at every set of positions the potential energy of a collection of atoms is defined. MD begins with the fundamental assumption that matter consists of atoms. The collections of atoms are treated as a mechanical system (moving with the potential energy). It is then possible to calculate the vibrational spectrum, thermodynamic properties, equilibrium structures, reaction rates and equations of state for the system investigated.

In quantum mechanics methods, electrons are included explicitly. In MD the electrons are not included explicitly due to the Born-Oppenheimer approximation (BO). This approach assumes that that it is possible to uncouple nuclear and electronic motion. In molecular mechanics it is considered that the electrons of the system find their optimum distribution. Chemical problems can be investigated considering the nucleus. Molecules are a collection of masses that interact with each other using almost harmonic forces. This is analogous to a ball and spring model, *i.e.* weights joined by springs. Positive increments are reflected by thermodynamically unfavorable contribution (distortions) to the molecule's potential energy.

The potential energy of the system is given as the sum of the potential energies of all the atoms involved. For each atom, a sum of energy terms (individual interactions that are a function of the coordinates). Parameters called force field and internal coordinates are often used. The force fields are often classified as bonded or non-bonded (non-covalent).

The function for molecular mechanics potential energy can be expressed as the sum of terms, which accounts for stretching of bonds, angles and dihedrals from equilibrium. There are also terms corresponding to sums over all pairs of atom pairs separated by at least three bonds. The electrostatic energy is calculated with a Coulomb potential. A 12-6 Lennard-Jones potential is used to calculate van der Waals energies.

In order to mimic the screening of electrostatic interactions by solvent both approximate (variations with distance) and more realistic (explicit ions and solvents) schemes can be used. Often the manner in which the parameters involved are derived determine the differences in the force fields. MD programs include GROMOS, CHARMM, AMBER, CVV, NAMD and others [559-563].

The ensemble method is a general statistical procedure for obtaining thermodynamics properties. The average of corresponding quantum state values with the same statistical weight yields the macroscopic thermodynamic properties introducing the concept of 'ensemble' of Gibbs. A great number of replicas (representing different values for positions and moments) of a system are characterized by several quantum/classic states but the same thermodynamics parameters. Thermodynamic properties obtained experimentally are represented by thermodynamic averages. The distribution of probability of the ensemble considered is used for sampling the configurations of the system.

Regarding the ensemble types, for fixed number of atoms (N), fixed volume (V) and fixed temperature (T) we have a Canonical Ensemble (NVT). For fixed number of atoms, fixed V and fixed energy E we have a Microcanonical Ensemble (NVE). For fixed chemical potential (μ), fixed volume and a fixed temperature (T) we have a Grand Canonical Ensemble (NVT). For fixed number of atoms, fixed pressure (P) and fixed temperature we have an Isothermal-Isobaric Ensemble (NPT). For fixed number of atoms, fixed pressure, and fixed enthalphy (H) we have an Isoenthalpic-Isobaric Ensemble (NPH) [564].

MD are widely applied and extremely versatile for studying biological macromolecules by doing simulations of the dynamics of systems of atoms. This is done using series of infinitesimal time increments and chosen force fields. From the potential energy function for all atoms of the system, it is possible to generate trajectories (time evolution of the molecular motion) of the molecular system by simultaneous integration of Newton's equation of motion.

Calculation of the gradient of the potential energy $V(r)$, yields F_i, the vector of forces acting on the i-th atom ($F_i = m_i a_i$, i-1,2,3.N) where m_i is the mass of each atom, a_i is the corresponding acceleration, and N is the number of atoms. The numerical integration of Newton's equations of motion is performed in minor steps (femtoseconds, *i.e.* 10^{-15} seconds).

Finite difference methods are often used in time integration algorithms. In these methods, the integration is partitioned into small steps (Δt). It is also expected to require little memory, be fast, duplicate the classical trajectory as closely as possible, permit usage of long time steps, be simple, easy to program, be time-reversible and conserve momentum and energy.

The Verlet algorithm [565] uses the accelerations (a) at time t, atomic positions (r) as well as positions from prior steps in order to determine new positions at time t + Δ. From Taylor series expansion we have r(t +Δt) = 2r(t) - r(t- Δt) + aΔt^{2}, *i.e.* the new position at t+Δ.

The Verlet algorithm, even with long time steps, yields good energy-conserving properties, are very compact and simple to program. Some disadvantages includes the fact that numerical errors are introduced and the awkward handling of velocities. Improvements of Verlet algorithms include the Beeman's algorithm [566] (better energy conservation and more accurate expression for velocities) as well as the 'Leap-Frog' algorithm (velocities are explicitly calculated) [567]. Typically, the directions of simulation in time of the methods are arbitrary, *i.e.* time reversible.

In order to increase the efficiency and stability of MD simulations various models are used. SHAKE [568], for example, can be used to reduce computer time as a constraint algorithm. Additional forces are assigned to the atoms maintaining bond lengths at fixed equilibrium values. It is thus not necessary to calculate stretching energies for frozen bonds. Simulations can be done for longer periods. With improvement of algorithms, the number of degrees of freedom decreased and the number of time steps increased. Other improvement in algorithms include RATTLE, SETTLE, LINCS, WIGGLE [569-572] and others.

Real size of most systems contain on the order of Avogadro's number (6.023×10^{23}) of particles. Despite great advances computers do not model more than millions of atoms at a time. Consequently, the size of the system is limited when MD is performed and only a limited number of particles are tracked. This can yield effects due to interactions of the container wall with the atoms.

Periodic boundary conditions can be used to eliminate surface effects by placing the system into periodic space filling shaped (cubic, rhombic, dodecahedrom and truncated octahedron) boxes whereas the simulation box is replicated infinitely through space (lattice). The periodic image in every box moves with the same orientation, as in the central box. Upon leaving this box, one of its images will enter through the opposite faces with the same velocity. The central box is a convenient coordinate system as there are no walls or surfaces. The number of particles (central box) in the entire system is conserved.

The most time consuming part of MD simulations are the non-bonded interactions. The potential functions calculations include Coulomb potential function and Lennard-Jones potential functions. Non-bonded interactions use a cutoff radius, which commonly does not exceed half the shortest box vector for grid search. This avoids interactions between particles and their images at the same time. Half the side length of the cell used for cubic simulations boxes.

Ewald sums and reaction-field approaches can handle long-range interactions (strong decay with distance). The Ewald interaction potential is the sum of a short-range term in real space and a Fourier space long-range term, which assumes an infinitely periodic system and specified by a dielectric constant medium

In the simulation box, the field on a dipole in the reaction-field approximation is divided into a cavity and a surrounding medium of electrostatic interactions summed explicitly in the cavity. The surrounding medium should be given a dielectric constant and act as a smooth continuum. Outside the cutoff sphere of atom/charge group, the medium is modeled as a dielectric continuum (specified relative permittivity) which modifies the Coulomb electrostatic interactions. The method yields polarization of the surrounding continuum and the reaction field on the molecule at the center.

Using a thermostat algorithm the NVT MD simulation is adequate to investigate the behavior of the system at a specific temperature (experimental conditions). One of the first MD thermostats is attributed to Anderson [573]. The desired T is replaced using a stochastic collision method in which Maxwell-Boltzmann distribution yields, randomly, the velocity of the particle. The method gives a distribution of energies of 'mini-microcanoncal' simulations.

For the thermostats algorithms of Berendsen (velocity scaling) [574], the system is coupled to a fixed temperature external heat bath whereas the velocities scaled at each step. Extended systems introduced by Nose and Hoover [575]. Berendsen and Parrinello-Rahaman [576] introduced common used barostats for pressure control in MD simulations.

MD simulations can yield mean square displacement of groups of atoms and velocity autocorrelation functions; analysis of energy components; including interactions between user-defined groups of atoms; root mean square deviations (rmsd) between a reference structure and a trajectory; complete rmsd matrix of a trajectory against itself or against another trajectory; analysis of the orientation of solvent molecules around solutes; radial distribution functions; rmsd of pairs of distances; hydrogen bond analysis; analysis of formation and breaking of bridges; chemical shifts; analysis of orientation of solvent molecules; ramachandran plots; positional root-mean-square fluctuations and radius of gyration of sets of atoms.

When entropic contribution and solvation effects among others are not considered, many demerits associated with scoring functions could be avoided *via* MD. It is possible to study effects of explicit solvent molecule as well as obtain different thermodynamic parameters (interaction energies, entropies, *etc*) using MD. This offers a widely applied computational method for investigating macromolecules. Although computationally expensive, there are numerous quite rigorous MD-based methods for determining binding affinities (free energy perturbation (FEP), thermodynamic integration (TI)) [364-366].

Effectively, MD can used to account explicitly for the effect of solvent molecules on protein-ligand complexes. However, for receptor flexibility it is more difficult in conventional docking. It is also used for refinement of experimentally derived structures. MD is now a well-established molecular technique. However although the core concepts in MD are now mature there is still continuous improvements in related innovations and improvements in force field models. MD is also supported by advances in high performance computing and graphic processor units making computational demands no longer a limiting factor.

Representative simplified MD approaches are Molecular mechanics/Poisson-Boltzmann surface area (MM/PBSA) method and linear interaction energy method (LIE). With a number of simple approximations, MM/PBSA and LIE can provide relatively good binding affinity at a moderate computational cost. MM/PBSA approximates binding affinities combining molecular mechanics and continuum solvent approaches with difficulty, however, to predict the entropic contribution to the binding affinity. LIE is a semi-empirical MD approach which assumes that the binding affinity can be extracted from simulations of the free and bound states of the ligand whereas, however, two MD simulations are needed, one for the complex and the other for free ligand in water. However, there is still absence of proven accuracy for guide lead optimization [364, 365]. Some of these topics will be discussed again in subsequent sections.

WATER AND SOLVATION EFFECTS

Water molecules and solvation effects are key components in influencing binding site dynamics as well as protein-ligand recognition. This is however difficult even at the quantum mechanical level, despite the chemical simplicity involved. It has been assumed that a strong binder should displace the water molecules present initially at the receptor surface and restored, subsequently to the bulk solvent. However, water molecules with multiple hydrogen bonds could provide enthalpy contributions out-weighing entropic cost of its immobilization [367-373].

Permanently bound waters can be identified whereas favorably bound receptor waters are not considered as unmovable since a ligand may still displace them. Bridging waters may be a by-product of crystalization conditions. Water molecules can be trapped in an energetically unstable position if it locks a favorable protein conformation.

Such waters that define highly druggable hot spots can be prioritized for desolvation when designing potent binders. There may be predictive improvement requiring however human expertise and intervention. Computational approaches can assess the impact of water molecules on ligand binding.

Pharmaceutical and manufacturing drug development spend considerable time to identify appropriate solvent to scale manufacturing. Desolvation penalty is important in drug design. There is a variety of models (explicit and implicit) to describe biomolecules in solution. When the problem is treated explicitly, electrostatic problems are investigated by averaging over a large number of systems configurations. In addition to two hydrogens and oxygen, the waters can also have zero mass charges to incorporate polarizability. Early models were used to reproduce quantitatively the properties of water. Some of these models use a parameterization for cut-off for long-range interactions whereas others used Ewald's summation to treat long-range interactions. Rigid water molecule models are used [577-582].

Implicit models have been introduced in order to reduce the computational cost involved in solvated simulations. Two basic types of implicit models have been introduced for implicit solvation. The models based on accessible surface areas (ASA) were historically the first. When simulation describes receptor and ligand immersed in a continuum (implicit) representation of the solvent we have a family of methods for investigation binding affinities (polar and apolar effects). In the implicit approach, the solvent is considered as a high dielectric continuum that is interacting with partial charges embedded in a solute molecule of lower dielectric constant. It is possible to model the solute response to the reaction field of the solvent dielectric by applying laws of classical electrostatics [577].

By solving the Poisson-Boltzmann (PB) equation it is possible to calculate the electrostatic solvation energy which is represented by the favorable interaction between a polar solvent like water and a charge. This contribution arising from the solvent in response to the charge is also called the reaction field. For simple spherical ions, the initial analytical expression obtained by Born is called the Born energy. Polar solvation is addressed in the fast but approximate generalized Born (GB) method.

Combinations of molecular mechanics (MM), solvent accessibility (SA), GB and PB yields the PB/SA, MM-PBSA, MM-GBSA methods. The GB/SA method, popular in biomolecular simulations, includes an approximation in the solution of the Poisson-Boltzmann equation for a system comprising the solute molecule immersed in a dielectric with counter-ions and also takes into account the loss of free energy due to the formation of a cavity in the solvent. It is a generalized Born model augmented with the hydrophobic solvent accessible surface area [577].

Continuum solvation models (CSMs) such as the polarizable conductor model (CPCM), the polarizable continuum model (CPCM), the conductor like screening model (COSMO) and the solvation models (SMs) have incorporated solvation effects into quantum chemical calculations. In these methods, a dielectric continuum solvent assumed outside a cavity is constructed around the solute molecule. The polarization of the continuum screens the electric field arising from nuclei and electron distribution. The surface charge density on the boundary represents the effects of polarization. The entire effect of dielectric polarization is described by screening charges arising on the interface. Cavity surface and solute describe the local system (problem) [578].

Non-polar contributions (hydrophobic effects), van der Waals interactions between receptor and ligand due to solvation and strain energies (conformation reorganization energy performed with full MM-PBSA method). Changes in solute entropy upon binding determined by single static structures or conformational ensembles. Single point calculations (SP/MM-PBSA), an ensemble of configurations or a combination of structural models, explicit solvent and MD simulations combined with continuum solvent models.

The LIE approach considers the linear combination of electrostatic and van der Waals interaction energies between environment and the ligand considering the free solvated ligand and the ligand bound to a solvated receptor. This approach can be used in combination with MD, MC/MD and energy minimization. It is taken into consideration hydrogen bonds between ligand and surroundings; accepted or donated, apolar, aromatic or polar ligand SASA; receptor SASA and ligand or receptor intramolecular energy; chemical functionality in the ligand as well a number of ligand rotable bonds [579].

COSMO-RS and COSMO-SAC are extensions of dielectric continuum-solvation models to liquid-phase thermodynamics, which requires input in the form of a molecule-specific distribution of the surface-charge density. The molecule placed in a cavity, with its exact size, within a homogeneous medium or solvent. The solvation free energy can be determined from the sum of the cavity-forming free energy and the charging free energy. The cavity-formation free energy is the change in Gibbs energy to form a cavity in a solution S of the exact size of the molecule. Charging free energy is the Gibbs energy to remove the screening charges from the surface of the molecule [578].

There is a wide range of solvation methods with varying sophistication, accuracy, computational cost and usage of implicit solvents. Explicit solvation incorporated in the molecular dynamics free energy perturbation (FEP/MD) which includes explicit solvent molecules in order to provide a realistic treatment of solvation with computational cost limitations. Some methods use mixed explicit/implicit solvent schemes. Other combination methods include quantum mechanics/free energy perturbation (QM/FEP), grand canonical Monte Carlo/Molecular Dynamics (GCMD/MD) schemes [580].

Multi-copy methods (MCM) places and minimizes many small molecule probes on the protein's surface in order to define the most important interactions. Multicopy simultaneous search (MCSS) is used to retain only the lowest-energy probes [581].

The continuum mean-field model describes electrostatic and non-electrostatic interactions between a molecule and the surrounding medium. The model combined with Hartree-Fock theory or density functional theory is used to describe the self-consistent-field polarization of the solute's electronic structure by a solvent [582].

It was recently presented a revised version of the water many-body problem denoted TCPE/2013, This is based on a static three charge sites and a single polarizable site, The protocol models the molecular electrostatic properties of water. Considering anisotropic short ranges, there is designed a many-body energy term to accurately model hydrogen bonding in water. The parameters involved reproduce, up to hexamers, the *ab initio* energetic and geometrical properties of small water clusters as well as the repulsive water interactions occurring in cation first hydration shells. It also reproduces two liquid water properties at ambient conditions, the density and the vaporization enthalpy. It reproduces several important water properties. The model appears thus to be particularly well-suited for characterizing ion hydration properties under different temperature/pressure/phases/interfaces [371].

Recent work (2014) has emphasized the importance of water in protein aggregation. Effectively, a currently very important problem, for treating protein-aggregation diseases and developing peptide-based therapeutics, is understanding the molecular determinants of the relative propensities of proteins to aggregate in a cellular environment. The authors report a crucial role of the surrounding water in determining the aggregation propensity of proteins both *in vitro* and *in vivo* [370].

SIMULATIONS OF FREE ENERGIES

We commonly characterize the interactions of most ligands with their binding sites in terms of binding affinities. They describe the strength with which a ligand, like a drug, binds to a receptor. The energy left once you have paid the tax to entropy is the free energy, which defines binding affinities. Enthalphy is the energy of interaction for a single binding pose orientation in the pocket. Enthalpy involves hydrogen bonds, polar interactions, van der Waals interactions. The sum over all possible poses in the pocket yields entropy (involves loss of degrees of freedom, gain of vibrational modes, loss of solvent/protein structure) [583-652].

The binding affinity is defined in terms of the strength between the ligand and protein interactions. The dissociation constant (Kd) is a measure of whether the interaction will be formed in solution or not. The binding affinity characterizes the binding of ligand and receptor molecules in solution. It is described by the molar Gibbs free energy which is related to K_d *via* $\Delta G = RT\ln(K_d)$ where R is the ideal gas constant and T is the temperature. The orientation of the ligand in a protein pocket is the binding pose. The interaction energy for a singly pose is the enthalphy. The sum over all possible poses is the entropy. Entropy is lower when a single pose is favored. A system (constant temperature and pressure) will evolve towards equilibrium in the direction of decreasing Gibbs free energy. For changes (ΔS) in entropy and changes (ΔH) in enthalpy we have ($\Delta G = \Delta H - T\Delta S$). There is a preference for lower potential energies. Thermal motion disrupts bond formation. The equilibrium between ligand A and its receptor B, as a phenomenon of association or dissociation, yields $\Delta G = RT\ln((AB)_{eq}/[A]_{eq}[B]_{eq})$. Ligands with high binding affinity require comparatively lower concentrations to occupy maximum sites.

Accurate values of ΔG are required for determining binding affinities (free energy simulations). It is necessary to probe the most populated states. Good quality potentials and population sampling is important. Free energy simulations yielding binding affinities is the backbone of a good description of ligand (drug)-protein interactions.

Lost/gain of free energies from changes (degrees of freedom (orientation, translation conformation), solvation effects, and ligand-protein interaction) yields subtle balances between energetic and entropic effects (changing entropies and enthalphies). Consequently, simulations of free energies plays a very important role in screening for lead drugs, calculating binding affinities and increasing our understanding of structure-activity relationships.

Classical statistical thermodynamics relationships connect the microscopic properties to macroscopic thermodynamics properties *via* canonical ensemble partition functions of the individual species, the complex and the solvent. The partition function enumerates possible microscopic states of the molecules. However, direct calculation of complex systems is often not feasible due to the configuration integral. Despite efforts to approximate the calculations *via* decomposition of the free energies, difficulties persist mostly due to errors in the calculations of free energy components. It thus becomes necessary to use empirically derived corrections or simplifying assumptions.

In the free energy perturbation method (FEP), the relative free energy of systems A and B is given as the ensemble average of the exponential (difference in energy of the two systems). This is divided by the Boltzman's constant multiplied by the temperature. To ensure satisfactory convergence, the two systems are connected by a reaction coordinate (λ). Simulations are made at multiple λ values for each pair of ligand investigated [586].

Thermodyamic integration (TI) uses the parameter λ (reaction coordinate, interatomic distance) allowing good space and phase overlap from systems A(reference state) to B (perturbed state). Simulations are made with varying λ values and calculations of the free energy gradient. This gradient is used to construct the potential of mean force (PMF) across λ [584,603-604]. In the FDTI method, small values of $\Delta\lambda$ are used to improve the overlap between the perturbed and reference states as well as the convergence of the simulations [589].

In the Replica exchange TI method (RTI), hamiltonian replica exchange moves are incorporated between adjacent λ simulations. This becomes periodic yielding exchanges between each configuration and its neighbor. Moves are rejected or accepted according to metropolis tests. Sampling is improved and simulations are able to move freely to configurations that are more favorable [587].

In the procedures of Adaptive umbrella sampling and adaptive umbrella weighted histogram analysis methods (ADuMWHAM) the parameter λ is treated as a dynamic coordinate which is moved throughout the simulation. The relative free energy is obtained from the potential of mean force along λ [317, 602].

In the parallel tempering (PT) method, multiple replica of the system is used to enhance sampling. Each replica runs at different temperatures. A Monte Carlo test is made with neighboring temperatures which can result in changes of the system' coordinates at these temperatures. Finally, a correct ensemble distribution is obtained from the set of trajectories at each temperature. The approach of PPTI (parallel tempering thermodynamic integration) uses different temperatures with replicas of the system. In this method, each replica runs at a different temperature [602].

Based on linear response theory, LIE is a linear interaction method. In this procedure, the compound's binding free energy is determined from the average of the potential interaction energy ensemble. The approach can use semi empirical, molecular dynamics and electrostatic models to estimate free energies between protein and ligands [604]. It can also be used as a scoring function.

Another approach to simulate free energies is the one-step (OS) perturbation method. In this procedure, rather than connecting A and B states by intermediate simulations, a single reference state does the work of sampling the degrees of freedom for both A and B states. Considerable gain is obtained if one state is chosen and used to calculate free energies for a series of end states.

The approach (LIE/OS) results from a combination of LIE and OS. One advantage of the combination is that the apolar contribution to the free energy is improved by the OS participation. Simulations of physically relevant states can receive most of the computational effort. The use of empirical parameters is reduced. Mostly, force-field description of the molecular system is required for estimating binding free energies [587].

In the approach known as λ-dynamics simulation, there is the propagation of the λ parameter with the atomic coordinates during the simulation process. The λ parameter is treated as a dynamic variable with a fictitious mass. Multiple ligands can be evaluated simultaneously. In the generalized ensemble TI method relative free energies can be obtained from a single λ-dynamics simulation. Trajectory snapshots can be sorted into bins and traditional TI equations used to compute changes in free energies [584, 585].

Constant pHMD is a variation of the λ-dynamics method, with the usage of fictitious λ particles to propagate titration degrees of freedom. In this method the end-states represent the protonated ($\lambda=1$) and deprotonated ($\lambda=0$) states. It is possible to incorporate in adiabatic free energy dynamics (λ-AFED) a λ parameter. Free energy profiles along reaction paths can be generated. Swithching functions generate high barriers between endpoints. Temperature and mass of λ are assigned [630, 631].

Multiple ligands that do not interact with each other are represented in multiple topology λ-dynamics representation. Biasing potentials are used as reference free energies. Restraining potentials added so that ligands do not go outside the binding pocket. The system partitioned into environment and individual ligands. The λ is treated as a dynamic variable linked to Monte Carlo variations after steps of molecular dynamics. The λ is also used as a self-regulating sampling variable to explore barriers and low-energy regions. It is also possible to associate λ values with multiple copies in order to sample regions of high energy. The λ-dynamics, however, have often focused on simulating difference at single sites in a given system [622].

In the path-integral method, a stochastic kinetic formalism is used to predict relative binding affinities of protein-ligand complexes. The ligand is modeled as a Brownian particle. The latter is subjected to nonbonding interaction potentials of the receptor allowing determination of relative binding affinities. Near the binding minimum, the diffusivity of the ligand and the curvature of the potential surface is used. These calculations are rapid and have given good results [586].

In nonequilibrium free energy methods (NE), λ incremented n times in the calculation (from o to 1). Here n is a constant for the calculation. Simulation sampling are allowed and summed between increments [629].

The free energy difference between two states is in principle equal to the work performed on the system. According to thermodynamics, this rule is for isothermal, reversible processes linking two equilibrium states. However, infinitely long processes are required for a switch (process linking two states) to be truly reversible. There are thus switching approaches in free energy simulations. In the switching method of Bennett's acceptance ratio (BAR) there are switches in backward and forward directions to calculate differences of free energies estimated from the lower bound of the average work. Other approaches improve sampling of the switches *via* weights for size and position of increments. In the method of bias sampling configuration, sampling is used for bias yielding increments of λ [628].

In the non equibrilium harmonic oscillator approach (HO) sampling is made in A and B systems with differing hamiltonians but the same number of oscillating particles. Many of the properties, including free energy differences are calculated analytically. This is useful for comparisons with correct answers [589].

There has been recent advances to construct biomolecular free energy landscape from a MD simulation. In order to reduce the large number of MD trajectory atomic coordinates, the method uses a systematic principal component analysis. The system is reduced to few collective degrees of freedom. The protocol uses internal coordinates (backbone dihedral angles in the dihedral angle PCA) to avoid artifact mixing of internal and overall motion. The procedure also makes the choice of an appropriate dimensionality of the energy landscape (containing all slow large-amplitude motions of the molecule/neglecting coordinates describing high-frequency fluctuations) [633].

Recent work reports the evaluation of the relative free energies of bio organometallic compounds. The method explores the conformational space by means of Molecular Dynamics simulations. It uses the semi empirical PM6 protocol coupled with the COnductor-like Screening MOdel solvation model followed by density functional theory (DFT) calculations. The DFT-D3 dispersion energy correction is included for the most stable conformers. The calculated structures and free energies are in agreement with those of the experimentally detected molybdocene-cysteine adducts [594].

The inability to quickly generate rapid/accurate/robust parameters for novel chemical matter limits the application of molecular dynamics simulations in drug discovery. It was recently reported the Force Field Toolkit (ffTK), which minimizes common barriers to ligand parameterization. The protocol uses algorithm and method development. It also uses automation of tasks. The procedure can generate quantum mechanical target data, setup multidimensional optimization routines and analyze parameter performance. Parameters are developed for a small test set of molecules in order to reproduce experimentally measured values for pure solvent properties and free energies of solvation [595].

Recent work reported free energy molecular dynamics simulations of stabilization of duplex DNA and RNA. Umbrella sampling free energy simulations of dangling cytosine and guanine nucleotides have been used to investigate the molecular origin of dangling end effects. Calculated free energy contributions associated with the presence of dangling nucleotides were in reasonable agreement with experiment predicting the general trend of a more stabilizing effect of purine *vs.* pyrimidine dangling ends. Both electrostatic and van der Waals interactions contribute to the duplex stabilizing effect of dangling end nucleotides. The free energy simulation scheme could also be used to design enhanced duplex stabilization [596].

QUANTUM MECHANICS/MOLECULAR MECHANICS METHOD'S

Semi-classical statistical mechanics and empirical or *ab initio* derived force fields can be used by atomistic methods to determine transport and thermodynamics properties. For large systems, molecular mechanics can be used. The force fields results from the fact that the total potential energy is differentiable with respect to atomic coordinates. Force fields can be determined for atoms. These can be used for simulations using molecular dynamics.

Semi-empirical methods use simplified version of equations from *ab initio* methods. They can treat valence electrons explicitly and include parameters fitted to experimental data. They are relatively computationally less expensive and can handle larger systems. It may be however sometimes difficult to determine the quality of the results.

From first principles, *ab initio* methods can solve numerically the quantum mechanics Schrodinger (or Dirac) equation to calculate exact properties from only the coordinates and species. This includes bond breaking/formation, chemical reactions and ligand-protein binding. The method is however computationally expensive and limited to small systems and fast processes. These calculations can be up scaled by using elastic tensors, diffusivities. viscosities and force fields determined for MD simulations. The *ab initio* methods can also be downscaled by fitting electronic integrals in semi-empirical methods [644-712].

Density functional theory was well received because of the high computational/scientific limiting demands of first-principle-based calculations. At a more computationally affordable cost, density functional theory (DFT) opened the way for more accurate calculations with larger models (more atoms).

The number of electrons or atoms determine the level of sophistication for the calculation. Starting from the lower level, we have the empirical potentials (10^1 to 10^6 atoms). Tight binding calculation (10^4 atoms). Higher levels of calculations includes self-consistent fields (SCF) Hartree Fock (HF), correlation perturbation theory, configuration interaction and DFT. On the order of $\sim 10^2$ atoms are used with SCF and DFT methods.

In the Born-Oppenheimer approximation, the electronic motion is decoupled from that of the nuclei. The many-electron wave function is in 3N dimensional space and the total energy is the expectation value of the Hamiltonian. Correlation is not included and computationally more expensive methods (configuration interaction and many body perturbation theories) had to be introduced.

It was observed that, as in condensed matter physics, the density can be used as a key variable. Systems should differ only by their potential energy. This would provide a versatile, viable alternative. In 1964 Hohenber and Kohn show that all many-body systems are a function of the ground state density and could be determined. DFT subsequently became one of the most popular tools in the theory of electronic structure. The genius of this work, involving this simple idea, was to realize that it allowed the original many-body problem to be replaced by an independent electron problem. This can be solved by requiring the ground state density to be the same as the exact density. We can divide the Kohn-Sham equations into one part for independent particles and another for the exchange-correlational function. The energy is minimized and eigenvalues are approximated to the energies. It is necessary to assume a form for the exchange correlation.

Density functionals have evolved through local spin density approximation, gradient-expansion approximation, generalized gradient approximations (GGA), Meta-GGAs, time dependent DFT (TD-DFT), hybrids, functionals to include (H-bonding, longe-range corrections, thermochemistry, barrier heights, transition-metal reaction energies, non-covalent interactions, valence and Rydberg electronic excitations, non-local correlation, intermolecular interaction energies in DNA, amino acid pairs and reaction energies in organometallic chemistry [653-712].

Recent developments in DFT includes (2012) the d-functional tight-binding (DFTB) method based on the d.-functional theory as formulated by Hohenberg and Kohn. The method introduces several approximations. First, the densities and potentials are written as superpositions of atomic densities and potentials. Second, many-center terms are summarized together with nuclear repulsion energy terms in a way that they can be written as a sum of pairwise repulsive terms. The Kohn-Sham orbitals are expanded in a set of localized atom-centered functions (represented in a minimal basis of optimized atomic orbitals). These are obtained self-consistently for spherical symmetrical spin unpolarized neutral atoms. The Hamilton only contains one- and two-center contributions which can be calculated and tabulated in advance as a function of the distance between atomic pairs. The method addresses self-consistent charge extension, weak interactions and a linear response scheme [656]. Using a Taylor expansion around the reference density the protocol has been extended to first, second (modification of Coulomb scheme) and third-order (new parametrizations scheme) models with applications to organic and biological systems [655, 656]. The modifications allegedly leads to improved overall performance [657].

QM/MM (quantum mechanics/molecular mechanics is an approach that can be used to approximate binding affinities. The basic premise is the combination of the strength of both QM (more accurate) and MM (efficient, faster) methods to generate a strong tool for investigation of systems (including biological) which are divided into two regions. The inner region is treated quantum-mechanically whereas the outer region can be described by a force field addressed respectively as QM and MM regions [366,374-380].

The ligand would be the QM region for a protein-ligand complex whereas the protein would be the MM region. Special attention needs to be paid to the boundary between inner and outer regions. QM/MM methods were originally used for modeling reactions in biological systems and gradually emerged as important tools for predicting biological activity of inhibitors. They indicate good correlation between computed interaction energies and biological activities of inhibitors. The model provides good potential to improve the interaction energy of the lead compounds with a reasonable computational cost [374-380].

SIMILARITY-BASED

Since structurally similar compounds can have similar biological and physiochemical properties, similarity-based VS have become an important part of *in silico* drug discovery. This protocol permits fast identification of biologically active analogues. However, adequate representation of the molecules involved is required. These representations include one-dimensional descriptors (log P), 2D descriptors (MACCS structural keys), 3D descriptors, spatial pharmacophores (CoMFA fields) [200, 239, 381-392, 458, 534, 537, 713-799].

The fingerprints calculated from a molecule's geometry, as with human fingerprints, may be sufficiently detailed whereas comparing two molecular fingerprints may be almost equivalent to comparing the molecules themselves [381-383]. VS often use the 2D fingerprint and 3D shape similarity methods.

These include MACCS, rapid overlay of chemical structures (ROCS), extended-connectivity fingerprints (ECFP) and phase SHAPE. It is also possible to use long bit strings to encode 1D or 2D projections of molecular topology including as well properties such pKa and logP. This can be complemented with additional structural descriptor information, such as shape recognition data for identification of active molecules.

The evaluation of docking methods is often based on their capacity to rank ligands data sets consisting of known binders (with corresponding decoys/nonbinders). It is necessary to pay attention to the physical properties of the compounds in the decoy sets in order to obtain a fair assessment. Let us define physical similarity as that among some physical properties such as (number of rotational bonds, molecular weight, log P (cLogP), number of hydrogen bond acceptors and donors). Let us also define chemical similarity to that involving chemical structure such as (functional groups and molecular topology). These can be measured using molecular fingerprints and Tanimoto similarity score. In most screening libraries there are differences in chemical as well as physical properties. Unfortunately the scoring functions used in docking sets can be undesirable influenced by physical properties of the ligand. This would result in bias of the screening results.

The performance of similarity-based methods can also be affected by the compounds structural classes. In these cases different approaches can generate different results and show little overlap in similarity relationships.

MOLECULAR FIELDS

The molecular recognition between a ligand (the drug) and a macromolecule (target) is a fundamental postulate in the classical drug design paradigm. H-bonding, stacking, ionic and hydrophobic interactions are often observed in ligand-protein interactions. Molecular electrostatic potentials are important. Interaction forces can have inductive, dispersive and electrostatic components [713-762].

Dispersion forces result from non-polar molecules (temporary dipoles in neighboring molecules) and induce fluctuations in electron distribution in neighboring systems. The interaction of polar and non-polar molecules yields inductive forces. Due to charges or permanent dipole moments, polar molecules yields electrostatic interactions. An atom or molecular fragment can be used to describe the variations of its interaction energy with that of a 3D molecular structure. This allows prediction of how and where ligands can bind to a biological target with improved activity [713-738]. Considering energy and shape simultaneously, Goodford [714] did pioneering work fitting ligands within the active sites of biological macromolecular targets.

Graphical energy contours (molecular interaction fields (MIFs)) representing the interaction probes (functional groups, molecules) with sample spots (at x,y,z coordinates) can indicate hot spots of energetically favorable ligand-target interactions. Nonbonded atom pair interactions can be detected by Lennard-Jones functions for attractive and repulsive van der Waal forces. Minimum distances between atoms needs to be established to generate attractive forces. Charges on probe and targets yields pairwise Coulomb electrostatic terms which takes into consideration the spatial dielectric medium.

Regarding molecular probes, they should represent the most important groups involved in the interactions. Often used probes are carbonyl oxygen and amide nitrogen probes (hydrogen bond donor and acceptor groups); hydrophobic probes (hydrophobic interactions). Probes are often parameterized spheres (specific ion or atom) with hydrogens treated implicitly. Nonspherical, multi-point, rotatable probes to find best possible hydrogen bonds can also be used.

The mapping of binding sites by MIFs can be useful in drug design. In CoMFA (comparison of molecular field analysis) [716, 717] differences of ligands with changes in intensity and shape of intermolecular fields around molecule are analyzed. In CoMSIA (Comparative molecular similarity indices analysis) [718, 719] hydrophobic fields, hydrogen bond donor, acceptors, and electrostatic features are considered. Similarity indices are calculated in the place surrounding each of the aligned molecules in the data set.

Grid molecular interaction fields can yield detailed information by highlighting the favored interaction sites and the type of interactions involving the target proteins. In the mathematical GRIND approach (Grid-Independent descriptors) descriptors are calculated independently of the orientation in space. The most important grid interactions as a function of distance are represented. This approach represent a class of alignment-independent three-dimensional molecular descriptors which are important for biological property description. Molecular interactions fields are simplified and encoded using autocorrelation transforms. The resultant molecular descriptors yields correlograms (graphical diagrams) used in chemometric analyses.

Using 'grid modes', analytic MIF expressions can be sampled over space surrounding the molecules at regular intervals. These method can yield hundreds or thousands of data points including 'hot spots' (regions of space with the most favorable energies (favorable binding sites). Algorithms can also be used to extract sets of hot spots from MIFs [723]. The node of the MIF can be tagged by the atom contributing most to the field energy. Energy cutoffs are used for node prefiltering making it possible to discriminate between weak and relevant nodes.

Grid MIFs are also used with high-throughput virtual screening of proteins. The binding site is first described and then fingerprints for ligand and proteins (FLAP) methods are determined and used to encode and compare the information. GRID-MIFs and GRID-FLAP methods are also used for identifying new targets. There are diverse methods that use MIFs to identify protein structure with high propensity for interaction with ligands [744].

3D molecular similarity measures used for matching groups of atoms *via* geometrical criteria can miss topologically different molecules that exhibit similar biological effects. Two molecules can have similar biological properties with different covalent structures and chemical formulae. Usage of molecular electrostatic potential (MEP) is a protocol that avoids limitations of atomistic models. Various field-based methods use 3d grids for comparing and sampling MEPs. It is noteworthy, however, that compared to other 3d-LBVS techniques, this can be computationally expensive. Global superposition can be misleading because of pitfalls in defining initial structural superposition as well as best overlaps in a specific region of interest [384-386].

MOLECULAR SHAPE

According to Frank Lloyd Wright in 1908, form and function should be one, joined in a spiritual union. Determination of molecular shape and changes in properties can be important for understanding the molecules involved in chemical reactions. Shape often determines the end-product as a result of molecular interactions with preferred and non-preferred biological targets [239, 797-804].

Enzymes can use shape recognition to differentiate between functional groups in a molecule. Shape recognition is also used by natural products (biosynthetic pathways) for selective oxidation. At the molecular level, chiral recognition involves mutually induced conformational adjustments. Ribozymes from *Escherichia coli* recognize cloverleaf-shape RNAs.

Chemical shape plays an important role in senses. These include olifactory receptors (smell), receptors for perception of color (sight) as well as taste. Addition of complementary electrostatic or steric interactions to molecular shape should increase specificity.

Life, survival, targeting molecules with bioactivity are result of the complementarity of binding in peptide-receptor, molecule-protein and antigen-antibody and protein-protein interactions. Shape can be important in ligand specificity, substrate recognition and antibody recognition *via* models of quantitative structure-activity relationships, docking, similarity-search and classification protocols.

Shape and shape-based descriptors can be useful molecular descriptors. One of the problems of molecular docking involves predictions of the pose within the active site of the receptor which is the result of hydrogen bonds, coulomb forces, hydrophobic interactions and van der Walls forces. However, geometric complementarity, apart from physical-chemical complementarity is not understated. Geometric complementarity is taken into consideration in various docking algorithms.

Among the state-of-the-art 3DVS techniques, molecular shape matching plays a significant role in protein-ligand interactions. Molecules that share similar 3d surface shapes are often assumed to likely share similar drug-like properties suggesting that 3d LBVS shape comparison techniques can offer a protocol for discovering novel drug leads. Due to important conformational changes (induced by binding), it may be desirable to generate a diverse ensemble of conformers [387-391].

Gaussian density functions are an efficient and elegant approach to represent and compare molecules. These can be first aligned with Cartesian coordinate axes by diagonalization of a second order steric multipole matrix, calculated from the atom-centered Gaussian functions. Subsequently, minimizing the sum of atomistic Gaussian overlaps can superpose pairs of molecules [392, 393].

Spherical harmonics (SH) functions can also be used for fast shape-based protein-ligand docking and virtual screening. These methods use SH polynomial expansions in order to represent the surface shape and other molecular surface properties. Subsequently, the special rotational properties of SH functions are used to perform fast Fourier-based correlations yielding efficiency in high-throughput receptor-based virtual screening [394-396].

BINDING SITE-BASED

In terms of physicochemical properties such as shape, size, hydrophobicity and polar interactions, all biological targets possess ligand binding pockets complementary to their ligands. The similarity of these properties in binding pockets for diverse proteins should lead to similarity of bound ligands.

This considered, it should be possible to apply, on a wide scale, computational approaches designed to detect physicochemical similar properties of binding pockets. This could also facilitate identification of potential off-targets as well as the whole multiple-target ligand design process [397, 398].

INVERSE MOLECULAR DOCKING

Potent binding of a small molecule ligand is not guaranteed by the presence of a protein-binding pocket. It is desirable to be able to directly predict protein-ligand binding complexes as well as their binding affinities.

Notably, although the general application of molecular docking is to search compound database for potential binders, there is no fundamental reason why molecular docking should not be also used to identify potential targets from a protein database for one small ligand.

Consequently, inverse docking protocol could be developed to dock compounds against databases of protein binding pockets using PDB structures [399].

Chemical Universe

If we consider small molecule, (mass less than 500 daltons) there could exist on the order of 10^{60} chemically distinct feasible molecules. This number far exceeds the size of any current compound database. The current bases do not surpass on the order of 10^8 inorganic and small organic molecules.

Since the sun is estimated to have 10^{57} hydrogen atoms, our theoretical chemical universe exceeds by far the possibilities of computer aided drug design. The ensemble of all known compounds does not represent even a very small sampling of the chemical universe.

It is thus clear that only a small fraction of the available chemical universe is explored in drug discovery [400, 401].

PROTEIN DOCKING

For living organisms, protein-protein interactions are essential since they are involved in most biochemical and biological processes, including redox reactions, signal transduction, protein transport and immune response. These interactions are of considerable biotechnological/therapeutic interest. They have potential applications for drug design (despite scarce complex formation experimental data). The combined importance and difficulty of protein-protein interaction prediction have stimulated research in this field [402-412, 750-788].

Protein-protein interactions can be defined as physical contacts between pairs of proteins. These occur in a particular biological context by selective molecular docking. They can be classified as: (a) interactions of protomers that cannot exist on their own *in vivo* (enzymes) and (b) interactions of protomers that can exist independently (antibody, antigen complexes). They are therapeutic drug targets and the mechanism of protein association is of considerable interest to drug discovery.

The two main problems of protein-protein docking methods are the following. The first is the 'conformational search' used to generate the correct conformation of the two proteins together. Target identification is the second most difficult problem. How do we recognize a native conformation among millions of generated configurations? The increase in computational power allows us to generate many configurations (including some close to the native conformation). It is noteworthy that the individual proteins can also undergo conformational change upon binding.

Scoring functions have been used to solve the problem of recognizing a native or near-native conformation (among millions generated). For the conformational search, most methods use a two-stage process. A rigid-bod global/local search is done in the first step in order to determine the relative position and orientation of the two proteins. In the second step there is account for side chain and backbone flexibility *via* refinement of the configurations. In the absence of information on the complex, fast Fourier transform (FFT)-based algorithms and geometric hashing can be used to identify binding modes. These approaches use grid point and scan the space by translating and rotating one grid about the other. A correlation-type scoring function is used to evaluate the docked configurations on a grid.

When geometric hashing is used, we describe the protein surface by critical points. These are used to detect geometric complementarity. Genetic algorithms and Monte Carlo (MC) simulated annealing are used to explore the potential regions. In these methods the search is confined to the starting structure. It may be possible to miss the correct conformation. Restraint-based docking can be used to direct the search.

Steric overlap is often included in the thousands of complex structures generated by rigid-body docking. Backbone and side chain refinements are subsequently required. One way to do this refinement is to use energy minimization (atomic force fields). Other approaches used include Montecarlo and genetic-based algorithms, multicopy, self-consistent mean field, principal component analysis and normal modes approaches. However, it is noteworthy, that if the conformational change upon binding is large, refinement may still fail to determine the native pose.

Many new technologies indicate that we are in a new research era of global biological systems. In order to understand a biological system at molecular levels it is necessary to identify and characterize the bio-molecular entities (proteins, genes). It is also necessary to build bio molecular maps indicating the relative location and movement, ways and paths with links and crosstalks [402-412].

Extraction of detailed information regarding proteins is made possible through the advances in imaging techniques. For drug design, creation/crystallization/imaging of macromolecular complexes is required. There are still relatively few protein complexes deposited in the Protein Data Bank limiting the growth of computational approaches (protein-protein docking) in this field. Effectively, in protein-protein docking it should be possible to determine the relative conformations and transformations of two proteins which yields available energetically stable/favorable complexes. It is possible to construct appropriate representations/correlations of two rigid proteins using the cumulative overlap of their electron densities. The search can be simplified using rotational angles and coarse grids and knowledge of binding sites. In the absence of this information, exhaustive sampling can be used to find minimum configuration. The calculations can be accelerated by using Fast Fourier Transforms and Spherical Fourier correlation based approaches.

As observed with protein-ligand interactions, discrimination between native and non-native poses are required for accurate docking predictions. A range of protein docking programs are available (ZDOCK, DOT, PIPER, RDOCK, MolFit). Scoring functions and their combinations are typically used [763-768].

ZDock use pairwise electrostatics, shape complementarity and pairwise potentials. DOT uses Poisson-Boltzmann electrostatics and van der Waals energy. PIPER uses a GB based procedure with shape complementarity. FRODOCK [768] uses van der Waals, electrostatics and desolvation correlation functions as well as spherical harmonics-based docking. Other programs use coarse-grained potentials/decoys.

Effectively the scoring functions use chemical properties, solvation terms, evolutionary conservation and shape complementarity. They can be divided into empirical, forcefield-based and knowledge-based. Compared to receptor-drug complexes, with concave/convex interfaces, the flat interfaces in some protein-protein interactions makes shape complementarity harder to detect.

Recent work reports a protocol that the authors suggest improves the state of the art in initial stage rigid body exhaustive docking search, scoring and ranking. Improvements are introduced in electrostatic affinity functions; shape-complementarity, novel knowledge-based filters, GBSA reranking procedure and a new knowledge-based interface propensity term with fast Fourier transform formulation. Algorithms including dynamic packing grids can be used to speed up the calculations with error bounds [788].

Targeting protein-protein interactions is an attractive new approach to drug design due to increasing available information regarding structures of protein complexes and signaling pathways. In this approach drugs must be designed that can specifically interfere with, for example, dimer and oligomer formations (multimer protein forms), cause disruption of antibody-antigen interactions (fast pharmaceutical segment) and alter a signaling pathway by targeting protein interactions [787].

Different approaches should be introduced since the binding sites differ from traditional small ligand-protein interactions. It is noteworthy, there are already various databases of protein-protein inhibitors. Nonetheless, for designing drugs to interfere with protein-protein interaction there are many challenges. Extensive databases of starting structures are required. The type of small ligands that comprise the traditional protein-ligand databases are inappropriate since typical protein-protein interfaces are approximately 750-1500 A^2. In addition, more shallow surface areas define protein-protein interfaces.

Effectively protein-protein interface flatness makes difficult the design of small molecules (blocking of interactions). Large number of scoring functions developed over the years for small ligands may be inappropriate. Protocols developed over the last decades for protein-ligand binding may not be effective for the challenges of finding small deep crevice-like binding pockets (enzymes or receptor ligands). Significant conformational change can be observed for proteins and their surfaces on binding to a partner. Protein-protein contact surfaces can be large and dominated by hydrophobic, steric, electrostatic and hydrogen bond interactions. The interfaces are flat, broad and large, often containing residues. One advantage is a strong contribution from hotspots.

Validated protein-protein inhibitors, machine learning and chemoinformatic methods have been applied yielding promising patterns and trends. These include the information that at the interfaces, many Trp, Phe Tyr and Met residues are present [782]. Lipinski's rule is not typically observed, since the inhibitors considered (with nanomolar Kds) have molecular weights of at least 650 KDa.

Typically, we expect broad/flat/large protein-protein interfaces. Noncontinuous epitopes are also compromised by contact residues. Despite the large interfaces, most of the free energy of binding is contributed by small hot spots. These sites can be prioritized as drug design targets. In some cases, fragment based ligand design has been successful for designing these ligands.

Protein-protein interfaces show adaptability, can change from the unbound to the bound state and are flexible. Created binding cavities not seen in the free protein can disrupt the protein-protein interactions. Motions of small loop perturbations and side chains often define the conformational changes. At interfaces, crevices/pockets can be accessed by small molecules. The crevices may not be accessible by the protein partner. For static structures of protein-protein complexes it is difficult to predict their disruption by small molecules.

For docking of inhibitors, NMR and 10 ns molecular dynamics simulations can be used to predict dynamics and flexibility in protein-protein interactions. Other methods include MM-PBSA, component analysis of decomposition of solvation energy, regression based scoring functions, normal mode analysis, coarse grain alternatives, hybrid MD/normal mode analysis, constrained geometrical simulations, and random walk rotable bonds. The multiple protein structure method (MPS) incorporates flexibility to identify hot spots using MD. Simulations of MD also used to study intramolecular conformational changes and water mediated hydrogen bonds [749-787].

Many machine-learning approaches have been also used in the last decade for protein interaction site prediction (Bayesian Network, Support Vector Machine, Artificial Neural Networks (classification methods) and Ramdom Forests, Conditional Ramdon Fields (sequential labelling methods). With the exponential growth of protein sequence data, an exploration of new methods that predict protein interaction sites based only on sequence information is becoming increasingly important. MetaPis is a recent sequence-based Meta-server for protein interaction site prediction [750].

Despite diverse difficulties involved, several dozen published inhibitors (small molecules) have been reported to disrupt protein-protein interactions [787]. This is quite promising.

Stem Cells

Stem cells are very special. They are able to differentiate and self-renew to somatic cells (mature) *in vitro* as well as *in vivo.* They differ in culture, longevity and variety of types they can generate. Induced or embryonic, the pluripotent stem cells are most potent. Adult cells are restricted in differentiation potential.

Stem cells' ability to generate relevant cells in limitless supply makes them biopharmaceutical attractive. Over forty years old, bone marrow transplantation is the most established. Other stem cell treatments have progressed to the clinical stage [413-417, 805].

The high cost and not well-understood regulatory pathways hampers the development of some therapies. There are also risks of transplantation of undifferentiated/malignant transformations. Alternatively, stems cells can be used in conventional small molecule drug discovery. Here we find well-established manufacturing/regulatory pathways. Somatic cells (stem cell derived) are alternatives to current recombinant cell lines.

It is now possible to develop disease-specific stem cells and rapidly generate panels with ranges of genetic phenotypes. Consequently, a more accurate prediction of how a drug will behave across a mixed population is possible. Another important potential application of stem cells lie in the discovery of regenerative drugs that could promote cells to repair lost/diseased tissues for cases such a heart failure and stroke.

Currently, difficulties in directing routinely stem cell differentiation *in vitro*, hampers development of their full potential. In addition, there are difficulties associated with high pure populations, high yield, large scale, reproducibility and cost effective challenges.

The study of disease progression and pathology *in vivo* should soon be routinely possible. This should be enabled by the ability to generate disease specific iPS cells (reprogramming adult somatic cells to a pluripotent state).

Current drug screening methods face many challenges/difficulties. They rely largely on usage of recombinant transformed cell lines that express the target of interest. The use of physiologically relevant primary cells is desirable. These are difficult to obtain and it is challenging to obtain sufficient numbers for high-throughput screening applications. There is also the problem of variability between donor and preparation of cell batches.

An attractive alternative is offered by stem cells, which can be propagated for prolonged periods, be cryopreserved and can differentiate to relevant cell types. Large batches of cells can be generated for use in experiments and screens. iPS cells can also yield disease specific somatic cells. They can yield panels of stem cells with different genetic phenotypes. Genetic effects on drug performance can be investigated.

HTS screens have reported cells differentiated into specific receptors and pharmacologically responsive to specific compounds. Lineage selection technology is then used. As cells differentiate, drug selection can be applied such that, all cells not expressing the resistance gene dies. This is a powerful technique for selecting, from a heterogeneous mix of differentiated cells, the lineage of choice.

Stem cells can be used to generate *in vivo,* models for a particular disease, which can be used in a drug screening campaign or investigating how a drug behaves in a particular disease. It is possible to generate cells for a variety of diseases differentiated to patient-specific somatic cells. Against these, Small molecules could be screened to see which could correct the underlying defect.

Cells can also be generated from patients with many diseases. Another challenge lies in the studies of complex neural diseases (Alzheimer's disease). In these cases it may be necessary to mimic the progression *in vitro* and obtain enough diversity to simulate the mix of cell types which are present and affected *in vivo*.

In addition to conventional drug screening, there is also interest in discovering novel drugs to promote repopulation lost or diseased cells (stroke for example). Alternative targets for screening are endogenous stem and progenitor cells that can themselves regenerate.

A large number of drugs fail in the early stage of clinical trials because of toxicity costing drug developers billions of dollars a year. Primary cells are expensive, in short supply and vary significantly from donor to donor. Pluripotent stem cells provide consistent limitless alternative resource for toxicity studies. This can considerable reduce the need for animal testing.

Reliably, robust and direct reproducibly to functional specific high yield cell types is an important requirement for the previously discussed applications. Novel protocols are needed to accelerate the usage of this technology. Novel approaches should include the usage of robotic high throughput platforms. Along these lines we also have the miniaturization of cell culture using micro fabrication technique enabling screening in parallel.

Effectively, from target identification/drug screening to toxicology studies, stem cells have the enormous potential to revolutionize the drug discovery process at all stages [413-417].

VIRTUAL SCREENING

Virtual screening (VS) involves rapid assessment of large libraries of chemical compounds in order to guide the selection of lead candidates (using computer-based techniques developed for drug discovery). There is an increasingly larger chemical space (expanded to more than millions of purchasable, bioactive compounds). VS yields (low false hit rates)/(good yields) such that synthesis and testing tasks are manageable [418-546].

The most extensively used VS methods are docking (1), pharmacophore (2), quantitative structure activity relationship (QSAR) (3), similarity searching (4) and machine learning (5). These methods can be grouped as follows: a) structure-based virtual screening (SBVS); *i.e.* docking of candidate ligands into a protein target followed by applying a scoring function to estimate the likelihood that the ligand will bind to the protein with high affinity; b) ligand-based virtual screening (LBVS) which applies computational descriptors of molecular structure, properties, or pharmacophore features to analyze relationships between active templates and compounds from chemical libraries [324, 418-456].

In the first method, (1), active compounds can be identified geometrically by docking to a pre-selected target site followed by binding configuration optimization and scoring (enabling the identification of novel active compounds with their corresponding binding modes). Comprehensive conformational sampling, adequate modeling of solvation and entropic effects as well as improvement of scoring functions can be used to address the methods limitation in modeling target structural flexibility.

The classical docking-based VS approach begins with the usage of a three-dimensional structure of the target protein. Subsequently, usage of docking software as well as compounds can be stored in databases (docked inside the target protein). Scoring functions can be used to analyze the docking results. The ligands that interact better inside the receptor are selected and the most representative subjected to binding assays or *in vitro* inhibition. Beyond the classical docking-based VS approach, there is also usage of docking software as the central core of more complicated approaches.

In the second (2) or pharmacophore method, active compounds are identified by matching molecules to an assembly of steric and physicochemical features for activity. This method complements docking by its ability to select active compounds of higher structural flexibility but is less effective in modeling detailed binding interactions. It is also sensitive to training datasets, quality of conformational sampling, multiple choices of features, molecular overlay, binding affinity estimation and anchoring point selection.

The third (3) QSAR method makes usage of statistically significant correlation between molecular structures and activities to identify active compounds. Specific sets of structural and physicochemical properties (descriptors relevant to activities) can be used to represent molecular structures. This model is dependent on representativeness of structure-activity data, concept compatibility, and influence of data outliers, starting geometry, quantitative relationships and multiple choices of solutions.

The fourth (4) or similarity searching technique measures the level of structural similarity to known compounds in order to identify novel active compounds. The technique uses methods such as molecular fingerprints, molecular descriptors and molecular structural similarity. The technique is effective and fast but limited however to requirements of structural or sub-structural similarity to known active compounds.

The fifth (5) method is a machine learning method, which includes binary kernel discrimination and support vector machines using statistical analysis of intrinsic correlations between activities and the structural/physicochemical profiles of known compounds. The objective is to identify the active from the inactive compounds. The technique uses statistical models to predict diverse spectrum of structural and physicochemical properties at high CPU speed useful for screening large libraries. The method depends on training set diversity and parameter ranges.

High demands on screening speed and low false hit rates are placed on virtual screening due to significantly large libraries involved. Consequently, VS methods are used in combination with each other and with constraints/filters. These include drug-like filters such as Lipinski's rule of five, rotable bond counts and solubility. Constraints/filters also include structural ligand-centered binding-site, binding-mode selection, and applicability domain in QSAR and excluded volumes in pharmacophore methods. Combination approaches involves methods that complement each other in screening speed as well as hit selection strategies to yield enhanced performance. The faster method can be used first.

We can also make a division of the three-dimensional (3D) virtual screening methods into three main groups with corresponding sub-groups as follows. Group 1 is 3D-LBVS, group 2 is SBVS and group 3 involves other 3DVS approaches. In the first group, we have the following: a) 3d fingerprint-based screening (alignment/comparison of molecular fingerprints); b) molecular fields comparison (superposition/comparison of molecular fields); c) ligand shape matching (superimposition/comparison of molecular surfaces); d) 3D-pharmacophore matching (screening for a ligand conformation matching pharmacophore); e) 3d-QSAR (information derived from the ligands conformational space).

Group 2 is SBVS and involves protein-ligand docking (exploration of the ligand conformations space); binding site similarity (comparison of simplified representation of macromolecular binding sites); molecular dynamics (whole target structure and ligand atomic-level properties).

Group 3 involves some of the other 3DVS approaches. It is subdivided in fragment-based VS (identification of small chemical fragments; chemogenomic (identification of novel drugs and drugs targets); knowledge-based drug discovery (data modeling and knowledge extraction).

Virtual screening methods have adjusted during the decade to screen, with promising performance, increasingly larger chemical libraries involving even more than millions of compounds. The continuous development of library generation tools requires still further improvement of virtual screening methods to meet the complex screening challenges. Effectively, further improvements of individual VS methods include consensus-modeling strategies, integration of VS and HTS, mining of actives and inactive from libraries, addition of off-target identification, side effects prediction, improving efficiency and productive performance of search methods. VS techniques require further improvements to meet the challenges [418-456]. There are numerous docking and virtual screening programs. Some of these protocols will be reviewed in subsequent sections of this chapter [492-546].

WORKFLOW PIPELINES

We refer herewith to more efficient virtual screening protocols. These are cyclic process with each cycle leading to more accurate data. This often involves applying hierarchy of filters of increasing selectivity in order to reduce rationally large virtual libraries to smaller sets of candidate molecules for experimental evaluation. The procedure uses fast filtering funnels first and subsequently more computationally expensive tools to distinguish remaining candidates [457-463].

Molecules can be first selected with good ADME-Tox properties and drug-like features in order to improve pharmacokinetics and potency. Subsequently, 2D or 3D similarity filters can be used for further screening followed by pharmcophore modeling to obtain desired structural chemical features. Further filtering involves docking with molecular dynamics in order to predict binding modes and optimize substituents. Lead candidates can then progress to stages of synthesis and testing and the results re-cycled through 3d QSAR and ADME-Tox prediction models.

Multiple levels of varying sensitive filters (ADME-Tox and scoring) can be used to scan very large libraries (hierarchical screening *via* combination of LBVS and LBVS methods). More advanced workflows management systems can be used to make the tasks accessible providing flexible frameworks to build complex workflows and analysis pipelines [457-463].

DIFFERENT TYPES OF LIGANDS/TARGETS/INTERACTIONS

For ligand-protein interactions, most docking protocols have been developed for traditional small organic molecules. There are however ligands/targets/interactions that merit special attention. We will comment briefly on some of these cases [789-811].

Hydrogen bonds interactions are mainly electrostatic soft interactions. They are dependent on the pair of atom groups that forms the acceptor donor subunits.

Their bond lengths and angles fluctuate according to local environments. Crucial for binding affinity/drug design they dictate the orientation in the receptor of the binding ligand. The vdW term is known to be the primary origin of the stabilization energy for stacking between aromatic rings.

The characteristics of halogen bonding are parallel with those of hydrogen bonding in terms of directionality and strength. This type of bonding can be important where the control of self-assembly and molecular recognition is important. There are many structures in the Protein Data Bank with halogenated ligands [790].

Boron (positioned just before carbon and nitrogen) has the potential to play an important role in medicinal chemistry. The usage of transition metal-catalyzed borylation reactions to prepare organo-boronates and the approval of Velcade (bortezomib) by FDA (for myeloma/lymphoma treatment) has contributed to borane chemistry. Boron compounds are in clinical and preclinical stages for treatment of various diseases including diabetes, inflammation and cancer [804].

The binding interactions between proteins and carbohydrates (most abundant biopolymers) are vital for life in nature. Both intrinsic protein-carbohydrate and extrinsic chaperone-mediated mechanisms are used for covalent attached carbohydrates in glycoprotein folding.

The immune system functions are directed by carbohydrates/carbohydrate-binding proteins on proximal cells. Most membrane proteins on cell surfaces are glycosylated with a variety of attached carbohydrate chains. Changes in their patterns are associated with cancer growth and metastasis formation. A better understanding of these processes could improve our ability to design/tailor/stabilize protein-based therapeutics [286, 791, 805].

Transcription is responsible for construction of proteins and replication produces copies of DNA. These vital processes can be targeted with the help of ligand-DNA small binding molecules which can interact with DNA *via* intercalation or minor groove binding. Intercalators with two or more fused rings forming a planar structure and minor groove binding often possess crescent-shaped structures that complements the shape of the minor groove [375, 806].

An increasing number of drug candidates (anticancer and antiinfective, immunosuppresive, antiarthritis) are based on transition metal compounds. Related drug discovery pioneering efforts were based on the cisplatin (famous metallic drug) analogues. Althoug the cisplatin primary mechanism action is based on DNA, it is much more complex than often described, since its molecular recognition by regulatory proteins can involve many paths and biochemical mediators [792].

Matrix metalloproteinase (MMPs) are a family of calcium-dependent, zinc-containing endopeptidases which are responsible for the tissue remodeling and degradation. of the extracellular matrix (ECM), including collagens, elastins, gelatin, matrix glycoproteins, and proteo-glycan. MMPs play a crucial role in invasion and metastasis, are upregulated in the majority of human cancers and are involved in various pathological conditions [807].

Metal ions such as Na(+), Ca(2+) and Mg(2+), are present in milimolar concentrations in the extracellular environment where they modulate binding of ligands to plasma membrane receptors. Various types of ligands, including peptide hormones and drugs, bind metal ions, in particular Ca(2+), in the lipid milieu where it is proposed that the metal ion-bound forms of ligands represent their bioactive conformations [808].

Inhibition of the metalloenzyme carbonic anhydrase (CA) indicates pharmacologic applications such as anti-convulsant, anti-cancer, anti-glaucoma agents as well as potential for anti-infective drugs (anti-bacterial and anti-fungal agents). Sulphonamides and their isosteres (sulphamates/sulphamides) constitute the main class of CA inhibitors (CAIs). From the enzyme active site they bind to the metal dithiocarbamates (DTCs) inhibitors, with similar action mechanisms.

Because of covalency, ligand binding to metalloproteins could be different from other proteins requiring appropriate docking protocols. When available and not computationally prohibitive, quantum mechanics-based methods should give adequate results. Grid-based methods, modification of flexible side chains, covalent docking of reaction intermediates, geometry optimization of binding site structures can also be used.

A number of neurodegeneracy diseases (Parkinson's, Huntingtons', lateral sclerosis, and Alzheimer') can be associated with misfolded and aggregated proteins and peptides in the damaged neurological tissues. More than half of the recognized neurodegenerative diseases are associated with specific protein aggregates. For central nervous system diseases, the association with specific proteins and forms of aggregations has therapeutic and diagnostic implications [809-811].

The number of Alzheimer disease (AD) victims is expected to reach 6 million by 2050. In AD there is abnormal formation of plaques (aggregated beta amyloid peptide deposits as well as intracelular neurofibrililary tangles). They consists of hyper-phosphorilated forms of the microtubule-associated tau protein. Current clinical therapy for AD is mainly treatment (palliative) targeting acetylcholinesterase (AChE) or N-methyl-D-aspartate (NMDA) receptor.

The classical 'one target, one molecule' protocol may not be effective for AD given its multifactorial nature. Recent developments are focusing on the multitarget directed ligand (MTDL) protocol (drugs are designed to address selected activities/targets). The idea is to develop mltifunctional agents capable of hitting different biological targets.

Lens opacification during ageing arises from progressive, gradual self-assembly of protein aggregates to produce light scattering. Investigating protein aggregation in these diseases is necessary for mapping pathophysiological events and development better therapies/diagnostic tools [809-811].

Metal organic frameworks (MOFs) have important application for the controlled release of drugs. Molecular docking approaches can be used with MOFs to distinguish good drug candidates for incorporation predicting the binding behavior of guest molecules in agreement with experimental measurements. Molecular docking techniques may yield fast screening of drug candidates for adsorption to coordination polymers (controlled drug delivery and/or environmental remediation) [464].

There has been considerable recent increase of information regarding integral membrane proteins (transporters, channels, GPCRs) which are major targets of drug design. Knowledge of their structures should provide important guidance to develop new drug leads. However, the protein is often of non-mammalian source. In addition, the structures are often only homologues or fragments of true receptors. They are typically strongly modified in order to enable crystallization. The X-ray snapshot is generally ambiguous with regard to the state of the imaged receptor and opaque to signaling processes. It is also not well addressed by a single image, the important feature of targeting small molecules to specific subtypes comprising families of closely related receptors. Currently, the structures do not yield the complete picture, the tools are still too crude to be convincing. It is difficult to determine strengths of specific noncovalent interactions. Recent publication reports high precision structural modifications enabled by unnatural amino acid mutagenesis in mammalian receptors expressed invertebrate cells. This allows detailed tests of predictions from structural studies. This protocol can provide evidence regarding ligand binding interactions as well as variations in binding among receptor subtypes [789].

Integral membrane proteins are binding targets of a wide range of pharmaceutical compounds playing important roles in cellular functions (transport of molecules across biological membranes). An example, the 18 kDa translocator protein (TSPO) is primarily located in the outer mitochondrial membrane and is an important drug target. It is implicated in apoptosis, steroidogenesis, immunomodulation, cancers, neuroinflammation and neurodegeneration as well as visualization of the progression of these conditions.

CLOUD, HIGH PERFORMANCE AND GRID COMPUTING

For providing large scale computational [465-478] infrastructure on-demand, cloud computing (CC) is a more recent but important approach. The resources can be provided online and accessed from anywhere. The approach functions as a Service, Platform, Software and Infrastructure model.

It also has measured service resource pooling, rapid elasticity, broad network access and on-demand self-service. It uses public, hybrid, private and community cloud deployment methods. Service Level Agreements (SLA) are provided (confidence, virtualization and pay-per-use model). By offsetting capital with operational costs, computational costs can be lowered.

Cloud computing may become the next generation data centre. However, more market oriented resource management could be of interest. CC offers client-awareness, automation and ease of moving services and data within the cloud. It is also a utility that is service-oriented where networking, data storage, computing cycles are end-products. Maintenance/administration falls under the responsibility of the vendor. The usage of CC is metered (charged only for consummation).

CC offer massive scalability (cost only limiting factor) with flexible allocation of resources which can be useful for managing spikes even for large parallel tasks. Regarding on-demand resources (extensibility), in real time, resources can be added sometimes automatically. Computer hardware can be shared. Virtualization offers abstraction storage devices and physical servers. Different operating systems run on the same hardware.

For directions of improvements. Cloud application programming interface is important. Unified interfaces can make it easier to switch between cloud vendors. Graphical user interfaces should be another way forward.

What are the differences between cloud and grid/high performance computing? Well, HPC (high performance computing) or cluster computing uses a set of homogeneous machines. These can be connected locally by dedicated low-latency high-speed network (Myrinet or Infiniband). Locally owned clusters can have processors connected by high speed interconnects [465-478]. They can yield better throughput than either grid or cloud models. One the other hand, there is the disadvantage of fixed with at most limited extensibility.

Grid computing comprises a heterogeneous network of loosely coupled computers acting in concert to perform large tasks. There is no requirement for homogeneity of computing devices in grid computing which can be spread over a geographically diverse area connected *via* different networks. Each node on the grid can be administered differently with a common software to communicate the results of each other to a central location. There are similarities between cloud and grid computing. The principal difference is the hardware virtualization in cloud computing. This difference may help furnish security by isolation. CC is also an inherent business model with improved usability.

Computer-intensive calculations can be solved using cloud, high performance and grid approaches. Effectively, hybrid technologies should furnish advantages of high performance, cloud and grid computing. Virtual library construction/screening, molecular dynamics simulations and quantum mechanical calculations can be performed using the afore-mentioned approaches.

The usage of cloud computing in molecular modeling for large-scale and data-intensive applications appears to be compelling (generation of combinatorial databases, analysis of huge genome sequencing/genomics projects, virtual screening of millions of compounds).

However, in order to perform cloud computing, many technical/tedious tasks needs performing (installation, launching, monitoring, and terminations). This expertise is often lacking and may be one of the reasons for the infancy of molecular modeling applications. There are not currently a corresponding large number of publications using the CC protocol. Front-ends still needs to be developed to facilitate user access.

Due to the emergence of virtualization and open source web protocols, encryption to increase confidence cloud computing is a growing recent phenomenon. However, data security and cost remains an issue for potential users. Cloud computing appears to be past the peak of inflated expectations for emerging technologies. However, nothing is perfect and backup plans need to me made as well as robust architected solutions in order to avoid vendor lock-in.

POST-PROCESSING

Some of the new protocols use poses generated from techniques including docking, scoring and virtual screening. Different procedures can be used to improve (post-processing) the accuracy of the generated poses. Some of these techniques include the following [42, 342, 356].

1) Structural filtration from experimental binding.

2) Interactions and visual inspection to repair deficiencies of scoring functions.

3) Decoy binding and protein structure models.

4) NMR-derived proximities of ligands to target surface.

5) Sets of docked poses to derive the interactions required for pose filtering taking into consideration the prevailing interactions in the poses and both the receptor and ligand sites.

6) Pose refinement by global optimization.

7) Automatic self-organizing map of poses.

8) Footprint similarity.

9) Comparative intermolecular analysis.

10) Free energy calculations.

11) Weighted-residue profiles.

12) MD and QM/MM simulation/minimization.

13) Multiple outputs and rescoring

CHEMICAL LIBRARIES

A number of commercial and public domain chemistry databases (containing from thousands to millions of compounds) are available. The use of collections of available compounds is a well-exploited strategy in virtual screening. One route is to use validated synthetic protocols and available starting materials to prepare collections of virtual compounds yielding rapid synthesis and structure-activity relationships.

It would be good if for each compound the following information was included: 1) ionization states at physiological pH, 2) enantiomers and tautomers. 3) conformers within certain threshold from global minimum energy. It may be also necessary to filter such computationally demanding databases [479-486].

Important aspects of protein-ligand binding interactions can be addressed by using pharmacopheres (from three-dimensional structures of proteins). Compounds that do not have importance for binding structural or molecular properties can be removed. In order to find new leads we can use pharmacopheres (encoding essential, key, conserved features) followed by workflows with a narrower selection. In order to search for selective features/profile (excluded volumes, less conserved portions of binding site, specific intermolecular interactions) we may need more crystal structures with specific ligand features.

It may also be important to evaluate ADMET, biological and physicochemical properties at an early stage in the virtual screening process filtering out compounds (with poor drug-like and unfavorable, pharmacokinetic properties). It may also be necessary to filter out interfering properties for *in vivo* and *in vitro* experiments, highly reactive groups, promiscuous compounds, poor solubility/ absorption/ permeation as well as interference with accurate biological activity).

Simple rules are available for drug and lead identification. Modeling of ADMET properties and pharmacological similarity will play important roles in chemical library design and screening. It is expected that future increased integration of ADMET properties in virtual screening will improve the quality of generated hits.

There is also increasing interest in predicting drug repositioning as well as multi target/off-target activities. It is necessary to provide a good comprehensive framework of pharmacological, chemical and biological information on drugs (small drugs in particular) for virtual screening. Removing from the libraries compounds with similar structures (differing by isosteric replacements, substituents) will increase their chemical diversity. In some cases, however, it may be necessary to restrict chemical diversity to specific classes of compounds.

It is noteworthy that undesirable ADMET properties and difficult synthetic schemes can hinder virtual screening follow-up procedures. Solutions/suggestions could include virtual synthesis, retrosynthetic schemes, diversity-oriented synthesis, biologically oriented synthesis, click-type assembly of ligands into the protein binding site. Using novelty and chemical diversity criteria for assembling compounds from fragments may help identify hits that possess enough structural novelty to warrant patentability.

It is of interest for workers to have available chemical information of compounds that can be synthetized from commercial building blocks as well as purchasable compounds (including websites of academia and industrial libraries). In order to perform virtual screening most of collections require some level of 'curation', Depending on the virtual screening routine, collections with 2D sdf files for example, need to undergo 'curation' by the users. We note that raw formats permit rapid handling of large chemical data. Most commercial vendors update regularly their chemical collections.

Applications of computational procedures to process chemical data and include required information for virtual screening entails database 'curation' steps. This provides standardization protocols for same chemical information/record. It is, however, a formidable task since collections can involve millions of compounds and substantial information with differing formats involved. Hardware/software may be required to manage/store/share the large data influencing setups/potential usage and molecular properties (including molecular descriptors, annotations).

3D generators, not conformation sampling, should be standardized. It may also be necessary to remove salts as well as co-crystalized small molecules that are not a part of the inhibition mechanism and may mislead computational results.

Another process is filtering to obtain selected range of pharmacokinetic and physicochemical properties and reduce clinic attrition of drug candidates, using for example Lipinsky's Rule of Five. On the other hand, unfiltered databases may yield useful scaffold information on families of ligands that interact well with specific targets and may be useful for improvement of pharmacokinetic profiles and binding affinities.

Another problem is format standardization and redundancy in merging databases from different chemical sources. Non-redundant repository and non-ambiguous identification of chemical entities is important (using elimination of superfluous information and compound recognition during the storage process). We can use conversion tools, *i.e.* algorithms that encode molecular structure information on string codes such as molecular hash codes. Taking into consideration duplicate information, using compound recognition, the files can be cleaned and standardized. A common chemical format such as multiple sdf files can be used.

For the development of novel bioactive compounds, stereoisomers can play an important role. Different enantiomeric forms can influence different roles. The treatment using commercial compounds can be delicate. The information is not often provided. This can lead to *in silico* recalculation of stereoisomeric forms creating mirror images and identification of stereogenic centers.

Working with molecules that have at least three stereocenters can double the size of database collections. The increased database size could be very dramatic if more than eight centers are considered and most collections consider only four centers. Some virtual screening programs can calculate these large numbers of centers on the fly. Calculations of all forms are necessary for pharmacophere screenings (when say, four sites are involved, stereomeric forms and chiralties may be recognized).

The ligand in the binding site may show different protonation states than at physiological pH. This information may be crucial in pharmacophore and virtual screening/docking methods particularly when the information is poor regarding the target at issue. Some databases give a range of pH at which the ligands are often protonated.

It is well known that tautomeric forms can influence the binding of a ligand to a protein. Different forms can yield different pharmacophere hypothesis in virtual screening. The absence of this information can result in incorrect information on compound recognition/binding.

Since the bioactive conformation is not necessarily the most stable conformation, when using shape-based or pharmacophore screening, compound sampling in databases can be important. This can be particularly true in virtual screening when we can determine very closely the conformation that the ligand will assume in a ligand-protein complex. It is not necessary to pre-calculate the conformations

done 'on-the-fly' by the software and are not included in public and free-access software. The calculations involved are complex/time consuming/ requiring large storage space/efficient sharing of data.

There are also controversial points regarding restriction of database's dramatic increase. How much study is required using diversified methods (distance-dependent, random torsional angle changes, normal modes and Monte Carlo minima, conformation generators) which may be only considered explicitly by few databases?

Database size increase is sometimes addressed by using compressed files from broadband capabilities yielding significant preparation speed-up with pre-calculated multi-conformation databases.

The global hit rate for the development of new therapeutics still indicates major failures in converting new ligands into drugs. This is often attributed to more difficult to predict ADMET profiles (toxicity, metabolism, excretion, distribution, absorption). It is important to discard virtual screened compounds with poor physicochemical/ADMET properties, even before experiments are performed.

Sdf files are not cheap for storing large information, inclusion of annotations and chemical information. The virtual screening on plain text formats can be parsed sequentially. This yields inefficient/time expensive or reduced parallel calculations potential. One solution is binary format files that can include more information that is chemical, store and organize large numerical data. Disadvantage of binary formats is that they are not readable with other software. They also offers challenges involving management, merging and tools for upgrading.

Of considerable importance are web servers of databases that may include facilities for display, substructure, preliminary searches, compound retrieval and physicochemical, pharmacokinetic properties. These are widely used to store and retrieve molecular data. There are free access and commercial servers (database management systems) that can optionally perform the following tasks. They can compress archive files libraries, perform re-filtering, improve visualization, do computational rescoring and perform deep analysis of molecular annotations during virtual screening pipelines workflows.

A more efficient management of the large volume of chemoinformatic workflows/procedures may require the usage of manager Pipelines in order to speed-up the discovery of new bioactive compounds. Depending on the purpose there are continuously new conceived computer-aided drug design procedures as well as databases with advantages and drawbacks.

Molecular docking can be rationalized as the exploration for accurate ligand conformations and orientations within a given biological target that benefits when using single conformer databases. This procedure reduces computational time in calculating conformers during the screening as well as the pre-parameterization of docking runs before virtual screening campaigns.

With the development of new software and crystallographic structures yielding adequate pharmacophore hypothesis, we are witnessing a rebirth, going back to several decades of pharmacophere modeling (allowing screening of millions of compounds in shorter times).

We note that pharmacophores are three-dimensional representation of molecular features needed for binding to a biomolecule. The ligand conformation plays an important role for the matching of ligands with pharmacophore hypothesis. It may be necessary to pre-calculate the probable conformational states of the ligands, taking advantage of ready-to-use databases or use online computational tools.

The usage of online tools could make it possible for the end-user to screen very large number of compounds, downloading and further analyzing only small hit lead sets. Another potential future trend lies in the virtual screening of molecules for which many companies offer synthesis-on-demand as well as molecules that can be easily obtained in a few steps of chemical synthesis (tangibles),

It is well known that the complete chemical space is about 10^{60} organic compounds making impossible the creation of a comprehensive database. There are not sufficient corresponding free *de novo* databases although billions of compounds have been already analyzed. These efforts are also blunted by the absence of accompanying chemical synthetic routes. It may be more useful to generate restricted *de novo* libraries for specific applications. It may also be of interest to generate web servers that allow fast computational generation of *de novo* libraries and estimate the inherent difficulties of synthetizing chemical compound and their synthetic accessibility.

In the last decades, chemical libraries have provided valuable resources for drug design, ready-to-use tools, reliable and comprehensible selection of compounds from free and commercial sources that are purchasable for further wet lab experiments.

From a computational point of view, a fine-grained model divides the populations into several subpopulations, each assigned to different processors or machines. Each population can only exchange information with other connected subpopulations. The master-slave model (genetic algorithm) assigns the populations to several subpopulations. These are subsequently assigned to different processors in order to enhance the computer speed. The coarse-grained model uses the concept of migration and island in order to exchange information between subpopulations.

The parallel computation models take into account both the computation resource and the architecture of the search algorithm. The focus is on how the chromosomes exchange and communicate information between the subpopulations in order to affect the search population.

Considerable effort is being investing in high performance computing in order to speed up the protein-ligand docking prediction search process as well as sampling methods to provide better initial seeds and end results. Cloud computing is a promising research area for docking predictions by enhancing the tremendous amount of computing and storage resources whereas the focus is on how to divide and dispatch search algorithm computations to computer nodes to improve performance.

An important problem for heuristic algorithms is the quality of solution and the balance of computation cost. Most computing nodes are not centralized for grid and cloud computing. For algorithm design there is also the problem of wasting time waiting for other slaves to finish their tasks. Another algorithm to get better protein-ligand binding solutions consists of using migration and pattern reduction operators to filter out the worst search directions.

The rate of future growth of chemical/biological/compound/target information is unpredictable. The present size of some of the databases is astonishing, containing 10^7 compounds. Despite duplicate entries and different types of molecular representations for the same compound, the number of compounds in databases is very large. Biological activity of the molecules is also very large, containing millions of compounds with activities against 10^4 targets. There has also been considerable growth for biological target information including candidate protein coding genes for therapeutic exploration [479-486].

CONFIDENCE AND THE FUTURE

It is important to understand the errors involved in calculating drug-protein interactions, *i.e.* energetics of drug discovery for pharmaceutical research. A hit lead (drug candidate compound) has micro molar concentration and nano molar activity. A drug lead should act in a realm perhaps less than 0.5 kcal/mol [487-491].

Compared to quantum mechanics, force fields are rather simple tools, approximations that allow forces and energies to be quickly calculated. Included are dihedral and torsion interactions, electrostatic and van der Waals interactions between atoms. Of the 6-12 Lennard-Jones equation (van der Waals interaction energy), the '12' repulsive term is supposedly a too severe computational convenience. The calculation convenience in the spherical shape of atoms approximation does not hold for tight contacts. Simple, convenient point charges which are atom centered, have their dependencies and error of fit. Complex/time/effort/calculation difficulties are involved and improved parameterization are required for more rigor in the approaches. The simple methods made it possible for us to move forwards with larger steps in reasonable time, despite being crude approximations. Determination of molecular structures can be obtained by force fields at a reasonable level. They are however, not so good in the determination of energies.

Lennard-Jones equations are used to calculate van der Waals interactions whereas parameters are determined for each atom type with joint interactions determined by combining rules. It is noteworthy that there is significant effect on hydration free energies for even small differences in Lennard Jones terms. It is also known that the electrostatic interactions are larger and can depend on our calculations of the dielectrics.

Point charges, often used, are approximations involving the electrostatic interactions between atoms. Models for traditional net atomic charges can be unsatisfactory for representing molecular electric potential for some systems. Small changes/perturbations of partial charges can yield significant differences in calculated free energies of binding or hydration. There is thus a difficulty in determining the errors in calculated electrostatic energies. It is even more difficult to estimate the errors in charge transfer.

Regarding intramolecular force field terms (bond stretching, angle bending) some molecules will have torsions that climb up the potential well. These can be complex and difficult to duplicate with analytical functions (yielding errors difficult to estimate). It is impressive how force fields can duplicate the conformation and structure of isolated small molecules *in vacuo* and how they drive molecular dynamics simulations to duplicate and maintain biological systems.

Actually, there are not too many ways to pack connected atoms (by strong bond stretching and angle-bonding forces). Although we can reproduce many aspects of bio molecular structure, the information is less than that for small molecule crystal structure.

What are the consequences of molecular conformations from MD simulations? Biological motions of proteins appear governed by a large number of multiple rotors and inter-atomic interactions. The minimum of a conformational well is easier to determine than its shape. The error in force field may not make it possible to determine energies at the precision we need.

Considering the simplicity, regarding quantum mechanics, force fields perform admirable. A good answer is one given with an estimation of confidence.

Knowing that the desired accuracy is not present in some models should spur more innovation and demand for more enhanced approaches and fundamental science. This could include data from experimentalist, human's expert eye and tailored scoring functions.

Regarding evaluation and standards, we should hope for some sort of 'good computing' certification for software that meets certain community expectations. For the future, a lot will depend less on the hardware and more on the software (providing error estimates and some indication of confidence).

It would be commendable for software to be able to estimate additional information such as diverse physical properties; provide available experimental results; experimental and predicted values of related compounds; required precision for applications; clustering of like compounds by docking programs; list of related compounds and sample availability; chemical, physical, biological properties and synthetic procedures.

We need to also develop software that are goal-oriented, *i.e.* that could help us make decisions. 1) Tell us if a model is able to yield accurate protein/drug interaction energies. 2) Anticipate whether the correlation will be poor. 3) Driven by few point of high leverage. 4) Inform whether number of descriptors are too large. 5) Predict whether we can obtain the required accuracy and precision. 6) Use conglomerate of approaches/expert systems/decision trees assembled towards our goals. 7) Include table of look-up pre-calculated values. 8) Request for expert intervention. 9) Inform when key data is not available. 10) Recommendations for further experiments. 11) Inform if needed models are already available 12) Yield precise calculations of physical properties from first principles. 13) Inform us of potentially unobtainable goals. 14) Show the route for more tractable goals.

We should not have over-expectations of what our methods can do. We should not leave to experiment and interpretation the evaluation of our success. As computer speed increases, we will be able to run larger, more complex quantum mechanical systems and perform simulations with longer/more realistic comparisons with experiment/obtain more data and better statistics in order to improve our scientific quests.

There will also be significant growth of interplay between theory and experiment as computational chemistry will indicate the need for more experiments and vice versa. It will also be necessary to have a simultaneous increase of users' knowledge in physics, chemistry, biology, computation and statistics [487-491]. It is a long road but we are on track.

DOCKING AND VIRTUAL SCREENING PROGRAMS

Molecular docking is a computational protocol that predicts conformation of a small molecule binding. In almost every drug discovery project that identifies a lead, molecular docking plays an important role. The procedure can also be used to analyze lead-target interactions. It is commonly used to screen virtually libraries of compounds in order to identify those compounds with potential to bind to a specific target. Molecular docking protocols achieve their objectives by computing fitness scores for generated binding conformations. The algorithm searches the space and identifies the conformation with the highest score as the predicted binding conformation. Compounds with highest scores are considered candidate target-binding compounds. A good scoring function is an important component and this is still a current challenge [492-546].

Drug discovery research often relies on usage of virtual screening (*via* molecular docking) to identify active hits in compound libraries. Effectively, virtual screening, using a variety of methods, has been successful in finding hits in drug discovery. One- (1D) and two-dimensional (2D) ligand-based approaches are on one end of the spectrum. They rely on knowledge derived form the connectivity information (one or more active ligands). These include 2D fingerprints, substructure matching and even text-based simulations. These are fast successful methods. The results depend however, on the similarity of active database compounds to the query. Docking is on the other end of the spectrum. These methods rely on physics-based scoring of protein-ligand complexes. On one hand it takes more computational time, but on the other hand it yields the opportunity to find new and diverse actives. These can be unrelated to existing active compounds. Between these extremes we have we have 3D ligand-based methods (pharmacophore and shape screening). These protocols use the information from active ligand and look for other ligands that match the 3D properties of a query molecule. Combinations of methods can also be used.

We subsequently review 50 docking/virtual screening protocols.

GLIDE originally developed by Friesner *et al.* is now available in the Schrodinger software suite (Schrodinger LLC) as a module. With geometries and properties of the binding site receptor, the program generates grids before starting the docking job. An exhaustive sampling in the ligand molecule torsional space is done to generate ligand-binding poses during docking which can be divided into four steps. The program employs, during steps one and two, a series of hierarchical filters to search for possible locations of the ligand on the previously prepared grids. This is done in order to generate plausible ligand binding poses *via* a coarse screening. The steric complementarities of the ligand to the defined binding sites are examined by the initial filters evaluating ligand receptor interactions with GlideScore. The ligand binding poses selected by the initial screening are, in the third stage, minimized with force fields *in situ*. A composite score is used at the last stage to rank the resulting ligand binding poses and select the ones to report by GlideScore. Internal steric energies as well as nonbonded interaction energies of the generated ligand binding poses are taken into consideration [492].

GOLD is another option for molecular docking and virtual screening. The method originally developed by Jones *et al.* is now released by Cambridge Crystallographic Data Center. Gold uses a genetic algorithm in order to explore the conformational space of the ligand taking into account the conformational flexibility of several selected amino acids residues of the protein. An initial population of ligand binding poses are randomly generated from the given three-dimensional structures of protein and ligand. Each individual of the population is assigned a fitness score based on its predicted binding affinity using implemented scoring functions (GoldScore, ASP, ChemScore). Ranking of all individuals is done according to their fitness scores. The entire population is optimized iteratively *via* migration operations crossover and mutations. Parameters control the genetic algorithm sampling procedure (Selection Pressure, Population Size, Number of Islands, Number of Operations, Niche Size, Migrate, Operator Weights, Crossover, Mutate) [493].

LigandFit, originally developed by Venkatschalam *et al.* is now implemented in the Discovery Studio software (Accelrys Software) as a module. The procedure used has two major stages. A cavity detection algorithm used in the first step to identify potential binding sites. The second step consists of fitting the given ligand to a specified binding site. A Monte Carlo conformational sampling procedure is used which is guided by a shape-based filter necessary to generate binding poses matching the binding site. The DockScore energy function is used to perform rigid body energy minimization on candidate binding poses. Further ligand binding poses can be evaluated using external scoring functions [494].

eHITS is an unusual fragment-based docking program which is based on individually docked fragments. The program tries to find a global optimum. First a grid is created inside the active site of the protein with equal spacing of 0.5 Å whereas the ligand is divided into rigid fragments connected by linkers that are flexible. Each fragment is docked independently to the active site at every possible place *via* geometrical criteria with a scoring for each case without discarding any fragments. Secondly, the hyper-graph detection algorithm matches rigid fragments that are compatible. The best-suited combination of fragments is chosen for further studies. Subsequently, there is an attempt by the algorithm to connect ligand fragments with flexible linkers in order to recreate the ligand structure. Then, in the given active site of the receptor, the energy minimization is performed with the possibility of rigid translation and torsion angles. Knowledge-based scoring functions are used to predict the ligand binding affinity [495].

FlexX is a traditional fragment-based docking tool whereas the choice of the fragment (ligand based) is the key step since it makes the ligand core responsible for principal interactions with the protein target. The database of torsion angles is used to generate different poses of a fragment that is considered as rigid in further steps. The selected fragment is placed in the active site of the protein and alignment procedure is attempted to establish favorable interactions. For docking of each fragment, steric distortions are removed and the interaction energy estimated. The procedure is repeated for other fragments of the ligand. The ligand is reconstructed in an incremental manner [496].

FRED input consists of conformers for each ligand for a two stage docking procedure (shape fitting and optimization). During the first stage, a 0.5 Å-resolution grid is used for placing the ligand. All atoms of the active site are considered, including hydrogen, *via* a smooth Gaussian potential. Three optimization filters are processed, *i.e.* refining of hydroxyl hydrogen position, rigid body optimization and optimization in the dihedral angle space of the ligand pose. For optimization, scoring functions are used (ChemScore, Gaussian shape scoring, ScreenScore) [497].

HYBRID uses both the structure of the target protein and the ligand bound to the active site to pose and score ligands. The program is also capable of using multiple conformation of the target protein if more than one crystallographic structure is available. The docking and scoring algorithms are similar to that of FRED [498].

SURFLEX, can be divided into two stages. An ideal ligand fitting to the binding site is done at the first stage generating protomol. Different types of molecular fragments (hydrogen bond donor group, hydrophobic group, bond acceptor group) are placed into the binding site of the protein with the orientations and positions optimized to form maximum interactions with the protein. Protomol is formed by assembling top-scored fragments. An incremental algorithm is used in the second step to find optimal binding poses of the given ligand. This is first broken into fragments with their conformations explored. There is subsequent alignment to the corresponding regions on the protomol evaluated by their steric complementarity to the binding site as well as binding scores. This yields a complete molecule generated by incremental construction from top-scored fragments or from a crossover operation combining intact molecules. Final binding poses submitted to *in situ* comformational optimization using binding scores computed by the Jain scoring functions [499].

TMFS is a novel rapid computational proteochemometric method called train, match, fit, streamline (TMFS) which proposes to map new drug-target interaction space and predict new uses. The TMFS method combines shape, topology and chemical signatures, including docking score and functional contact points of the ligand, to predict drug-target interactions [500].

DARC is a structure-based computational docking approach using Ray Casting for carrying out virtual screening by docking small-molecules into protein surface pockets that can be used to identify known inhibitors from large sets of decoy compounds. It can identify new compounds that are active in biochemical assays. DARC can be used on Graphic Processing Units (GPUs) resulting in a speed-up of approximately 27-fold over those with a CPU alone. It enables screening larger compounds libraries, more conformations, and inclusion of multiple receptor conformations yielding enhanced screening results [501].

SeeDS, is another approach to fragment based drug discovery (structural exploitation of experimental drug start points) which includes the design of a fragment library and identification of fragments. These bind competitively to a target by ligand-based NMR techniques and protein crystal structures to characterize binding. Fragments that bind are then evolved into hits, either by growing the fragment or by combining structural features from a number of compounds [502].

AutoDock Vina is a program for molecular docking and virtual screening that uses a sophisticated gradient optimization method in the local optimization procedure. The calculation of the gradient gives the optimization algorithm a 'sense of direction' from a single evaluation and by multithreading. Vina can also speed up the execution by taking advantage of multiple CPU cores [503].

EADock was designed focusing on both accuracy and flexibility. The accuracy is achieved by using a multi objective evolutionary algorithm (combining two physically sound scoring functions based on the CHARMMM22 force field with an innovative sampling engine with several deterministic operators). The program is able to modify the force field to cross energy barriers. The flexibility is obtained by using CHARMM as a molecular mechanics engine [504].

SLIDE searches for geometrical and chemical similarity between the ligand and binding-site template defining favorable interaction points with atoms of the protein surface. The program uses PDB files of the active site of the target without hydrogen as well as mol2 files of the ligand. The active-site residues are not truncated allowing side-chain rotations for induced-fit modeling as well as a dense mode for generation of interaction points that is an unbiased construction of the template. The SlideScore empirical function can be used to generate solutions for docked ligands [505].

EAISFD is a computer assisted *de novo* drug design method, which combines the design engine EA-inventor with a scoring function featuring the molecular program Surflex-Dock. The method uses tagged fragments. These are preserved substructures in EA-Inventor. They are also used for base fragment matching in Surflex-Dock (constructing ligand structures under specific binding motifs). A target score mechanism is adopted that allows the method to deliver a diverse set of desired structures. The method can be used to design novel ligand scaffolds (lead generation) or to optimize attachments on a fixed scaffold (lead optimization) [506].

PythDock is a heuristic docking program that uses Phython programming language with a simple scoring function and population based search engine. The scoring function considers electrostatic and dispersion/repulsion terms. The search engine utilizes a particle swarm optimization algorithm. A grid potential map is generated using the shape information of a bound ligand within the active site. The searching area is more relevant to the ligand binding [507].

CAPRI implements a comprehensive suite of docking algorithms which were incorporated into a dynamic docking protocol consisting of four major stages. The first stage is a biological and bioinformatics research aimed at predicting the binding site residues. This is to define distance constraints between interface atoms and to analyze the flexibility of molecules. The second stage is rigid or flexible docking. This is performed by the PatchDock or FlexDock method, which utilizes the information gathered in the previous step. In the third stage symmetric complexes are predicted by the SymmDock method. In the fourth stage there is flexible refinement and reranking of the rigid docking solution candidates. This is performed by Fiber Dock clustering and filtering the results based on energy funnels [508].

VoteDock uses a consensus algorithm attempt to combine different docking approaches into a single and powerful prediction method. A set of representative conformations are selected from each docking algorithm to efficiently inspect different guided search algorithms for correct conformation of a protein-ligand complex [509].

SKATE is a docking prototype that decouples systematic sampling from scoring in order to improve docking accuracy. It systematically samples a ligand's conformation, rotational and translational degrees of freedom, as constrained by a receptor pocket, to find steric allowed poses. Efficient systematic sampling is achieved by pruning the combinatorial tree using aggregate assembly, discriminant analysis, adaptive sampling, radial sampling and clustering. Because systematic sampling is decoupled from scoring, the poses generated by SKATE can be ranked by any published or in-house scoring function [510].

CRDOCK is an ultrafast docking and virtual screening program that contains a search engine that can use a variety of sampling methods and an initial energy evaluation function. It uses several energy minimization algorithms for fine-tuning the binding poses. Different scoring functions ensures the easy configuration of custom-made protocols optimized depending on the problem at hand. A pre computed library of ligand conformations is used. It is initially generated from one-dimensional SMILES strings [511].

LigenDock is the docking module of Ligen which is based on two programs, *i.e.* a docking program called LigenDock based on pharmacophore models of binding sites, including a non-enumeraive docking algorithm. The accompanying module LiGenPocket is aimed at the binding site analysis and structure-based pharmacophere definition [512].

FIREDOCK is an efficient method for refinement and rescoring of rigid-body docking solutions whereas the refinement process consists of two main steps. In the first step there is rearrangement of the interface side-chains and adjustment of the relative orientation of the molecules. The method accounts for the observation that most interface residues that are important in recognition and binding do not change their conformation significantly upon complexation. The second stage involves side-chain movements, which are restricted, and thus manage to reduce the false-positive rate noticeable. In the later stages of the procedure there is smoothing of the atomic radii allowing for minor backbone and side-chain movements increasing the sensitivity of the algorithm [513].

GENIUS docking system enables induced fit docking (changes both conformation of the ligand and coordinates of the receptor to consider the flexibility of the receptor). It combines ensemble docking to use the conformation cluster of the receptors. Soft-docking (flexibility of a receptor is considered by changing the repulsion term of the protein ligand interaction in scoring functions, such as the Lennard-Jones potential term) is used to set the coefficient for every atom of the receptor and to relax the collisions between protein and ligand atoms. Evaluation of the ligand-binding mode can be made by the GENIUS Score. After a number of iteration steps it yields the predicted protein-ligand complex [514].

BetaDock approach solves the docking problem by putting the priority on shape complementarity between a receptor and a ligand whereas the approach is based on the theory of the β-complex. From the Voronoi diagram of the receptor (with topology stored in the quasi-triangulation) the β-complex corresponding to water molecule can be computed. The β-shape with the complete proximity information among all atoms on the receptor boundary is defined by the boundary of the β-complex. Pockets are computed where ligands may bind from the β-shape. The ligand quickly placed within each pocket by solving the singular value decomposition problem and the assignment problem. Taking as initial solutions the conformations of ligands within the pockets, genetic algorithms are used to find the optimal solution for the docking problem [515].

ParaDockS is a framework for molecular docking with population-based metaheuristics. The approach is the combination of an optimization algorithm and an objective function that describes the interaction. The software is designed to hold different optimization algorithms and objective functions. An adapted particle-swarm optimizer is implemented and the objective functions are the empirical p-Score and knowledge-based potentials [516].

DockoMatic is a high throughput inverse virtual screening and homology modeling tool (free and open source application) that unifies a suite of software programs within a user-friendly graphical user interface (GUI) to facilitate molecular docking experiments. Users can efficiently setup, start and manage IVS experiments through the GUI by specifying receptors, ligands, grid parameters and docking engine. This yields automatically the required experiment input files and output directories. The user can manage and monitor job progress and a summary of results is generated upon job completion [517].

MedusaDock is a flexible docking approach which models both ligand and receptor flexibility simultaneously with sets of discrete rotamers. The program has developed an algorithm which builds the ligand rotamer library 'on-the-fly' during docking simulations demonstrating a rapid sampling efficiency and high prediction accuracy in both self- (to the cocrystallized state) and cross-docking (to a state cocrystallized with a different ligand). The latter mimics the virtual screening procedure in computational drug discovery [518].

LigDockCSA is a protein-ligand docking software which uses a powerful global optimization technique, conformational space annealing (CSA) and a scoring function that combines the AutoDock energy and the piecewise linear potential torsion energy [519].

bhDock is a blind hierarchical docking method which uses two-step algorithms. It starts with a comprehensive set of low-resolution binding sites determined by analyzing entire protein surface and ranking by a simple score function. Subsequently, ligand position is determined *via* a molecular dynamics-based method of global optimization starting from a small set of high ranked low-resolution binding sites. Refinement of the ligand binding pose starts from uniformly distributed multiple initial ligand orientations and uses simulated annealing molecular dynamics coupled with guided force-field deformation of protein-ligand interactions to determine the global minimum [520].

NEURODOCK does automated docking of flexible molecules into receptor binding sites by ligand self-organization *in situ*. It was developed for the analysis of potential binding poses of structurally complex flexible ligands [521].

ICM methodology proceeds with internal coordinates in order to optimize, in a grid-based receptor field, flexible ligands. The potentials of the grid includes hydrogen bonds, electrostatic, hydrophobic and van der Waals terms. ECEPP/3 force field and MMFF partial charges are used to calculate energies. Global optimization begins with random conformational change of angles, free bonds and torsions according to the biased probability Monte Carlo algorithm. This followed by local energy minimization of the analytical differentiable terms [522].

DOCK in its original algorithm used a geometric matching algorithm to address rigid body docking in order to superimpose the ligand onto a negative image of the binding pocket. Force field scoring and on-the-fly optimization subsequently introduced. Some releases incorporated improved matching algorithms for rigid body docking as well as algorithm for flexible ligand docking. Subsequent versions use the DMS program to generate a molecular surface for each receptor. SPHGEN utility can be used to create the negative image of the surface. SHOWBOX generates a receptor box centered on the ligand and GRID utility can be used to pre calculate the scoring function potential grids [523].

MCDOCK carries out molecular docking operations automatically allowing for the full flexibility of ligands in the docking calculations. The scoring function is the sum of the interaction energy between the ligand and its receptor and the conformational energy of the ligand. In this program, the Monte Carlo simulation method is implemented to search for the global minimum whereas the final scoring function is the detailed atomic interaction energy based upon molecular mechanics [524].

RosettaLigand uses a sampling methodology to simultaneously optimize protein backbone, protein side chain and ligand degrees of freedom. Energy functions and algorithms used for stochastically exploiting protein and small molecule conformations whereas the function consists of van der Waals, hydrogen bond, implicit solvation terms as well as empirically derived torsional potentials. The docking algorithm consists of gradient based minimization and stochastic Monte Carlo moves. There is a pre-enumeration of major ligand conformations, subjected to torsion space minimization during the simulation. For all receptor side-chains. the rotamers in the binding site are optimized simultaneously using a simulated annealing procedure. The receptor backbone is allowed to minimize subject to restraints [525].

Q-DOCK^{LHM} is a method for low-resolution refinement of binding poses provided by FINDSITE^{LHM}, a ligand homology modeling approach. In addition to the pocket-specific contact potential derived from weakly related template structures, the program uses position-specific anchor restraints imposed on the predicted anchor binding modes. These are derived from weakly homologous ligand-bound template structures identified by threading. Upon global superposition of the threading templates onto the target's structure the top ranked binding sites are clustered. Subsequently, each cluster of ligands is used to detect the anchor substructure. Equivalent atom pairs are projected onto ligand functional groups and the anchor substructure defined as the maximum set of conserved functional groups. The average pairwise RMSD for anchor functional groups is calculated. The consensus anchor binding mode and its structural conservation is then incorporated in the Q-Dock^{LHM} force field [526].

SODOCK uses optimization algorithm based on particle swarm optimization (PSO) for solving the flexible protein-ligand docking problem. In order to improve efficiency and robustness an efficient local search strategy is also incorporated yielding an optimization algorithm for obtaining docking conformations of ligands with good scores for solving highly flexible docking problems. The method is a hybrid of particle swarm optimization and a local search. The algorithm is a population-based search model inspired by social behaviors of organisms such as the flocking of birds and is supposedly simple and quick to converge [527].

3D-RISM-Dock is a fragment-based drug design protocol whereas the numerically stable iterative solution of conventional equations includes a fragmental decomposition of flexible ligands. In solvent mixtures of arbitrary complexity, the flexible ligands are treated as distinct species. The computed density functions for solution molecules are obtained as a set of discrete spatial grids that uniquely describe the continuous solvent-site distribution around the protein solute. Potentials of mean force derived from these distributions define the scoring function for an automated ranking of docked conformations [528].

FIPSDock is a molecular docking technique driven by fully informed swarm optimization algorithm and adopts energy functions suite for solving flexible protein-ligand docking problems. The particle swarm optimization (PSO) optimization has been introduced to solve the conformational sampling problem. It is a population-based search algorithm for solving continuous nonlinear optimization problems intending for simulating social behaviors of organism such as a bird flock. In the canonical PSO algorithm, the velocity of the particles updated depending on the position of the global best particle and the best position. The unique feature of FIPS is that the particle communicates and uses information such as velocities and positions from all its neighbors rather than just the best one. The docking scoring function uses an updated suite with more accurate calculations of electrostatic contributions and desolvation energies [529].

MOLDOCK is an implementation of a variant of the evolutionary algorithm (EA) whereas computational approximations of an evolution course called genetic operators are applied to simulate the permanence of the most positive features. When there are many different possible candidates each option is ranked based on a set of scoring or fitness functions. The best ranked solutions are kept for the next iteration with the cycle being repeated until an optimal solution is found. This solution is the one with best scoring function, closest in principle to the crystallographic structure. To perform positional searches there are two biological inspired algorithms. One is a simplex evolution algorithm (SE) MOLDOCK SE. The other is the MOLDOCK Optimizer based on GDEA that is based on an EA adjustment called differential evolution (DE) which provides a distinct method for selecting and modifying candidate solutions (individuals). In addition to re-docking a procedure called 'crossdocking' can be used to further validate a docking protocol, in particular when several crystallographic structures are available. Procedure involves docking a number of ligands found in a variety of crystal structures of a protein identical to a single rigid protein crystallographic conformation [530].

LENsRD applies conformational selection theory to improve crossdocking efficiency. The protocol aligns more closely with the emerging picture of binding generated by conformational selection theory. The protocol uses pregenerated conformational ensemble to simulate ligand flexibility. The ensemble includes local minima of the ligand that are within 5.0 kcal/mol of the global minimum and generated by a thorough sampling of the potential energy surface of the ligand. Generated conformers are then minimized to produce local minima. This conformational ensemble is then rigidly docked with postdocking minimization in the active site [531].

VinaMPI facilitates multiple receptor high-throughput virtual docking on high-performance computers (leadership-class computing resources), using a large number of cores to decrease the time-to-completion of the screen. It is a massively parallel Message Passing Interface (MPI) program based on multithreaded virtual docking programs and used to distribute tasks. Multithreading can be used to speed-up individual docking tasks. It uses a distribution scheme in which tasks are evenly distributed to the workers based on the complexity of each task defined by the number of rotatable bonds in each chemical compound. In can handle efficiently multiple proteins in a ligand screen. High-throughput inverse docking is allowed [532].

PBVS+DBVS a structure-based pharmacophore (SBP)-guided method was suggested to generate comprehensive pharmacophores of a number of crystal structures of target-inhibitor complexes. It is a hybrid protocol of a virtual screening method, comprised of pharmacophore model-based virtual screening (PBVS), rigid and flexible docking-based virtual screenings (DBVS). The Protocol is used for retrieving new inhibitors from commercially available chemical databases [533],

Grid-based FPS is a grid-based molecular footprint comparison method for docking and *de novo design*. It is a multigrid implementation of the footprint similarity (FPS), scoring function (useful for identification of compounds that binds to a protein on a per-residue basis). The method is faster than its Cartesian-space counterpart that is good for on-the-fly docking, *de novo* design or virtual screening.It is used to tailor construction of new molecules to have specific properties [534].

Forecaster is platform for drug discovery that fully integrates computations, virtual, theoretical and medicinal (experimental, intuitive) chemistry to take advantage of the full potential of these approaches. It is a web-based platform and a number of programs (Prepare, React, Select) with the objective of combining medicinal chemistry and computational chemistry expertise in order to facilitate drug discovery and development. It specifically aims to integrate synthesis into computer-aided drug design. The platform is used to build virtual combinatorial libraries, filter and extract a highly diverse library from databases and dock them to receptors (fully automatically and done by computational chemists for use by medicinal chemists). It yields large enrichment factors and a high percentage of active compounds recovered [535].

3d-QSAR+CoMFA+CoMSIA+FlexX-Dock is a protocol for predicting competitive inhibitors. 3D-QSAR was built and validated based upon known inhibitors by means of comparative molecular field analysis (CoMFA) and comparative molecular similarity indices analysis (CoMSIA). The FlexX-dock program is employed to screen the database against the desired target. The 3d-QSAR models predicts from the virtual hits, the inhibitors with activity within the desired range. The protocol combines ligand-and structure-based approaches being capable of identifying new hits with topologically diverse scaffolds [536].

H-DOCK is a fast protein-ligand docking algorithm based on hydrogen bond matching and surface shape complementarity. First a divide-and-conquer strategy enumeration-based approach is used to rank the intermolecular modes between ligand and protein maximizing their hydrogen bonds matching. Each docked conformation of the ligand is calculated according to the matched hydrogen bonding geometry. A simple but effective scoring function, reflecting mostly van der Waals interactions, is used to evaluate the docked conformations of the ligand. For flexible docking, the rigid docking procedure is repeated for multiple conformations of a small molecule (ranking all together). Authors suggest that hydrogen bonding and steric hindrance can grasp the key interactions between ligand and protein [537].

GalaxyDock is a protein-ligand docking program with flexible protein-side chains. It accounts for the flexibility of preselected receptor side-chains by global optimization of energy based functions trained for flexible side-chain docking. The energy function is a linear sum of protein-ligand, intraligand interaction energy and intraprotein energy. The receptor is treated as rigid and the conformational sampling is based on conformational space annealing (global optimization). A fixed number of docking conformations referred to as a bank is generated and evolved until convergence [538].

QXP-BMD is a multi-step docking procedure for systems involving ligands composed of extended chains in their molecular structure and as thus displays difficulties because of torsional flexibility. The method addresses ligands with a high degree of rotational freedom in order to predict orientation and conformation within the protein-binding site. Starting from an initial full Monte Carlo docking experiment, this is achieved by performing a series of successive multistep docking runs using a local Monte Carlo method. This has restricted rotational angles, by which the conformational search space is limited [539].

BEAR determines a binding estimation after refinement. It is a fast and automated post-docking procedure that benefits either from the efficient conformational sampling of docking poses (*via* molecular dynamics) and of more accurate predictions of binding affinities (*via* MM-PBSA and MM-GBSA). Each protein-ligand complex emerging from docking is submitted to energy minimization. A multi-step molecular mechanics/molecular dynamics simulation protocol is used. This consists of an initial minimization of the entire complex, followed by short molecular dynamics in which only the ligand is allowed to move as well as final re-minimization of the complex. The final structure of each refined complex is used to estimate the free energy of binding (with MM-PBSA free energy predictions). Large collections of structures sampled during molecular dynamics are used. Satisfactory results are achieved with a single energy-minimized structure [540].

DynaDock is a molecular dynamics-based algorithm for protein-peptide docking including receptor flexibility. A docking procedure is used in which slightly overlapping poses are sampled in a first, broad sampling step. The obtained ligand conformations are subsequently refined using soft-core-based algorithm, optimized potential molecular dynamics (OPMD). The parameters are optimized with respect to the systems energy at each step of the simulation. The approach consists of two sampling and one final scoring step. In the refinement step, the poses from broad sampling are used as starting structures. After refinement, all systems are energy minimized and finally the refined poses are ranked using a specially optimized interaction energy-based scoring function [541].

CONSENSUS-DOCK is a customized version of the Dock4 program in which three scoring functions (DOCK4, FlexX and PMF) and consensus scoring have been implemented [542].

MOE multidisciplinary integrated platform and available source code provides flexibility to a wide range of scientific researchers. It is an all-in-one molecular modeling and visualization tool that is easily integrated and customizable. Users can add new functionality or make changes to existing algorithms. It contains a suite of pharmacophore discovery applications used for fragment-, ligand- and structure-based design projects. Pharmacophore modeling generates and use 3D information to search for novel active compounds, particularly when no receptor geometry is available using a generalized molecular recognition representation and geometric constraints to bypass the structural or chemical class bias of 2D methods. Ligand- and Structure-Based Query Editor Construct queries with an easy-to-use interactive query editor using either proteins or ligands (which can screen a conformational database to determine candidate active compounds that satisfy the pharmacophore model). It can customize pharmacophore annotations with SMARTS chemical patterns and Boolean expressions. It can also restrict shape (receptor or ligand) with volume constraints and refine the query with directional vector constraints, centroids of atoms, or partial matches on annotations. Active site analyses tools help identify key interactions of molecular recognition. Automatic Pharmacophore Generation and induced molecular alignments (from a collection of input compounds (possibly with activity data)). All possible discrete geometries and all possible combinations of feature query expressions are considered, enforcing limits on feature counts. Score queries are based on known active compound coverage, statistical activity enrichment and atomic overlap of matching conformations. Protein Ligand Interaction Fingerprints also automatically generated from bound ligands given a set of aligned complexes (or docking results). It rapidly screens a conformational database for compound conformations that satisfy a pharmacophore query. It searches multiple databases, a sub-range of molecules or a database of docked compounds. Partial matches, SMARTS patterns, output of all symmetric matches and specification of essential features are supported [543-545].

Molegro Virtual Docker (MVD) is an integrated platform for predicting protein-ligand interactions. Molegro Virtual Docker handles all aspects of the docking process from preparation of the molecules to determination of the potential binding sites of the target protein and prediction of the binding modes of the ligands [546].

RECENT EVALUATIONS, VALIDATIONS AND BENCHMARKING

In 2009 Cross *et al.* [812] published their work on comparison of several molecular docking programs for pose prediction and virtual screening accuracy They used 68 diverse, high-resolution X-ray complexes based on mean ROC AUC and ROC enrichment values for 40 protein targets in the Directory of useful decoys (DUD). The analysis indicated general trends in accuracy that are specific for particular protein families. Modifying basic parameters in the software yields significant effect on docking and virtual screening results. Expert knowledge is important for optimizing the accuracy of these methods.

In 2009 Li *et al.* [813] published an evaluation of the performance of a number of molecular docking programs on a diverse set of protein-ligand complexes. The top-ranked solutions produced by the programs were compared to the native ligand binding poses observed in crystal structures. Results are less sensitive to the starting structures for docking. As expected results produced by the programs at three different computational levels reveal that their accuracy are not always proportional to CPU cost. Binding scores of top-ranked solutions are in low to moderate correlations with experiment (binding data). The programs are less capable of handling flexible ligands and relatively flat binding sites. The programs have different preferences to hydrophobic/hydrophilic binding sites.

In 2010 Mukherjee *et al.* [814] used a 780 ligand-receptor database and reported docking validation of protein family and ligand flexibility experiments. The objective was to evaluate accuracy of docking protocols for regenerating bound ligand conformations and provide easily accessible community resources for development of improved procedures. Family based success is largely independent of flexibility. There is a strong dependence on binding site environment. There is a family-based analysis for rapid identification of good trends, bad trends, failures, scoring and sampling.

In 2011 Yuriev *et al.* [815] published a review on computational docking in which they concluded that flexibility and successful scoring remained significant challenges. Single input conformation could decrease docking accuracy. However, multiple ligands cannot guarantee accuracy. Dependence of input speciation is also contradictory. Structure validation should be taking into account. Superior algorithms and scoring functions may be more important than considerations of stochastic *versus* systematic methods in conformational analysis. Although consensus scoring seems to make a difference, the matter is still under evaluation and debate.

In 2011 Plewczynski *et al.* [816] published their evaluation of seven commonly used programs using the PDBind Database. They independently compared the ability of adequate posing (root mean square deviation) of predicted conformations *versus* the native conformations. Scoring was also evaluated by calculating the correlation between docking score and ligand binding strength. A wide range of different protein families and inhibitor classes was covered (more than 1000 protein-ligand pairs). It was observed that although the ligand binding conformation could be identified in most cases there was still a lack of universal scoring function for all types of molecules and protein families.

Verdonk *et al.* in 2011 [151] investigated docking performance of fragments and druglike compounds [151]. Comparison studies are not straightforward (produce conflicting results). Possible reasons include ligand and target types used, quality/resolution of targets, workers level of experience, preparation of ligands and binding sites. No correlation was observed between potency of ligands and docking. However, docking performance is better for ligands with higher ligand efficiency (form higher quality interactions with receptors).

Consistent and objective comparisons are required [817] which requires adequate test sets for each case (affinity or pose prediction).

A road to improvements for many state-of-the-art docking programs is the accuracy of the scoring functions (differentiation between active and nonactive ligands). Many scoring functions can be influenced by physical properties of the ligands. This bias involving physical properties can cause ligands with specific physical properties to incorrectly score better than others. Normalizing molecular docking rankings using virtually generated decoys were recently reported [818].

In 2012 a compendium of papers was published in volume 26, issue 6 of JCAMD. This work focused on most widely used docking programs which were evaluated for pose prediction/VS performance/strategies for improvement.

In 2013 Yuriev *et al.* [342] published their review on latest developments in molecular docking. There are established programs as well as new docking programs and their innovations (proposed to deliver improvements to address shortcomings of existing methods). There is not however, an unambiguous confirmation of claims better addressed by benchmarking studies.

Comparisons of different programs are generally performed using scoring and docking to identify best poses and binding strengths of ligands in binding cavities. No consistency was observed in terms for which scoring/programs/functions performed better. The task is conflicting and not straightforward. This is due to the types of ligands, targets, quality of target structures, practitioner's level of experience, preparation of ligands, binding sites as well as other differences in protocol.

For consistent objective comparisons development of appropriate test sets/decoy sets are necessary. As expected, the main conclusions support the fact that pose prediction in contrast to affinity estimation, is performed well, by existing programs. For specific target types, each program performs better than the other. This is probably due to poor scoring across the board. Good pose prediction does not correlate necessarily well with good scoring.

Challenges remain regarding prediction of binding affinities, effective scoring and proper sampling of ligands and receptors. When available, receptor flexibility is still far from perfect. Side chains and backbones should also be considered. It is possible to use multiple receptor configurations simulating target plasticity. However, smaller ensembles with appropriate ligands should work better (in comparison to MD-based or large experimental ensembles).

Induced-fit docking/homology modeling should produce good targets. Common emerging themes include system dependence on the effects of receptor flexibility, ligand enumeration and inclusion of specific water molecules. Target-specific functions and approaches are recommended.

The authors suggest that receptor and ligand sampling should be solved in the near future. With increasing computational resources, efficient new algorithms should be achieved. Scoring is a more difficult problem since we are dealing with entropy and more refinement is required for configuration terms.

We have to deal with solvation. Although specific water molecules can improve prediction, a very careful selection is necessary SASA may not work effectively in all receptor types since it does not account properly for electrostatics but it does however improves predictions. Only marginally better than scoring functions, the MM/GBSA and MM/PBSA models yields only modest correlations with experimental binding free energies.

Numerical scoring functions may have now reached saturation. New approaches are needed. A better understanding of ligand-protein interplay translated into better scoring is necessary for a breakthrough in the field of docking.

CSAR (Community-structure-activity resource exercise) in 2010 was a major development for docking and benchmarking scoring and docking programs (www.csardock.org). It was a novel approach for addressing field problems in a community-wide fashion. With the objective of collaboration *versus* competition, it provides high-quality public datasets for method development and testing for computational chemists in order to determine what is achievable.

Carlson and Dunbar's editorial appealed to the community to use resources in developing new algorithms, donate data, participate and develop methods capable of designing inhibitors at picomolar and nanomolar levels. In 2010 the first scoring exercise took place for gauging the state-of-the art for docking and scoring with diverse/large sets of complexes. With correlation to experiment (R^2) ranging 0.12-0.58, 19 different methods were submitted although no advantage for any type of scoring function was observed.

Badly and well scored complexes had ligands of the same size although properties (torsional and hydrogen bonding) varied significantly. It was suggested that improvements in scoring should come from minimization of complex structures, explicit account for water molecules, protein flexibility, more thermodynamic accurate methods for calculating free energies of bonding, target-specific scoring, curaton of dataset entries, paying attention to noncovalent interactions and chemical features.

The publicly released 2012 Community Structure-activity resource (CSAR) data set contains 508 compounds with known affinity values, 757 compounds with provided SMILES strings, 57 compounds with an available protein-ligand crystal structure, 185 compounds designated to be inactive. The compounds affinities, which span six protein targets, are given in different units of measurement from different assays. The data set provides the separated ligand and protein in their native bound conformations, the complex compound and a set of unbound ligand conformations [819].

The data sets were recently used to compare selected knowledge-based and force field based scoring functions. The knowledge-based component seemed to improve binding mode predictions. Scoring experiments, with full set of 2012 CSAR benchmark, indicates that without the knowledge of native protein and ligand conformations it is challenging to predict affinities and binding modes.

The van der Waals scoring functions perform much better on native protein and ligand conformations and can be used as a reference for scoring comparison. For binding affinity predictions, the use of pregenerated ligand conformations seems to lower the success rates much more than the use of non-native protein conformations. There is a smaller difference for binding affinity predictions. This may be due to the usage of side chain flexibility mainly for protein conformational changes. Future trends involve usage of side chain rotamer sampling and on-the-fly ligand conformational sampling.

The objective of SAMPL is to test protein and small molecule modeling. It is a 'blind' assessment (methods applied to data not seen by participants). Ideally, blind tests helps avoid the tendency to bias our theories and approaches to known answers. It is conceived as an opportunity for groups to test their methods, learn from the experience and share lessons learned. The objective of SAMPL4 is to build a series of successful blind challenges for computational chemistry (hydration free energy, host-guest, binding free prediction components) http://ccl.net/chemistry/resources/messages/2013/01/28.007-dir/index.html.

Critical assessment of predicted interactions (CAPRI) (http://capri.e.bi.ac.uk) is a forum (conducted every other year since 2001) for evaluating methods for computational (protein complex interaction prediction) and protein-protein docking. Groups are invited yearly to test their computational methods and predict the structures of protein complexes (experimentally solved and made public that year).

Some of the protein-protein docking computational methods that have competed in Capri include the following.

AutoDock (autodock.scripps.edu)

DOT (http://sdsc.edu/CCMS/DOT/

3dDockSuite(http://sbg.bio.ic.ac.ud/docking/)

Fiber Dock (http://bioinfo3d.cs.tau.ac.il/FiberDock).

BiGGER (http://centriafct.unl.pt-ludi/bigger.html).

KFC Server (http://kfc.itchell-ab.org/).

SymmDock(http://bioinfo.ed.cs.tau.ac.il/SymmDock/)

PI2PE(http://pipe.scs.fsu.edu/meta-ppisp.html)

DOCK/PIE;DOCK(http//:clsb.ices.utexas.edu/dock-by-pic/

CNS (http://cns-online.org/v1.3/)

ATTRACT(http//:www.t38.physik.tu-muenchen.de/08475.htm)

LZerDProtein-proteinDocking (http://kiharalab.org/proteindocking/)

GRAMM-X
(http://vakser.bioinformatics.ku.edu/resources/gramm/grammx)

Hex (http://hexserver.loria.fr/)

ClusPro 2.0 (http://nrc.bu.edu/cluster)

SurFit (http://sysimm.ifrec.osaka-u.ac.jp/surFit/)

CNS (http://cns-online.org/v1.3/)

ARIA (http://aria.pasteur.fr/)

HADDOCK (http://haddock.chem.uu.nl)

In order to identify druggable 'hotspots' of a binding interface for a protein-protein complex there is CastP server (http://ftmap.bu.edu). The objective of the method is to design compounds that bind to the intermolecular interface region.

Regarding performance of virtual screening methods we note that there are various performance metrics used. NSQ_AUC is similar to AUC. It is also based on the calculation of the area under the ROC curve [819, 820].

LogAUC computes the ideal area under the semilog ROC curve. It weights preferentially early enrichment. The method can be compared across different size databases and different active/inactive ratios. Nonetheless global metrics often outperforms early enrichmet methods.

Regarding crystal structure as a validation benchmark we note the following. Although crystal structures are often used in evaluation benchmarking and validation it is noteworthy that there is a wide variety in quality of crystal structures deposited in the PDB (validation tool and resolution structures). In addition to ligand coordinates, it may also be necessary to use experimental data (R-factor) for docking validation. In addition, it may be of interest to consider an ensemble of structures (different tautomeric, protonation states, stereochemistry, conformations) [821].

Regarding benchmark bias in decoys we note the following. The sets can have limitations due to restricted physicochemical similarity, small synthetic feasibility and restricted number of decoys. On the road for improvements it may be necessary to use on-the-fly generation of decoys, multiple decoy sets, increase feasibility for any active and matching properties between actives and inactives as well as virtual decoy sets. For time and resource efficient target-dependent evaluation of docking programs, the creation of tailor-made decoy sets for given sets of actives and inactives may be important.

The usage of high performance, grid and cloud computing, previously discussed is another route for improving docking and virtual screening outcomes. The usage of these protocols are indicating increasing scale-ups and speed-ups of both individual dockings and virtual screens.

SELECTED APPLICATIONS OF VARIOUS MODELS TO DRUG DESIGN

During the last decade, we have applied many of the methods discussed in this chapter to Cancer, Aids, Diabetes, Alzheimer, Parkinson and other diseases.

In 2002 we made a theoretical *ab initio* study of ranitidine We used the HF and MP2 methods in order to investigate the open and folded ranitidine conformations and found good agreement with experimental crystallographic data. Our results suggested that, as in metiamide, the folded conformation is also preferred. We investigated electrostatic, hydrogen bond, solvent effects and charge distributions on stabilizing the conformations. The interactions of ranitidine with the biological receptor was discussed [1].

In 2003 we investigated nucleoside analogs that inhibit human immunodeficiency syndrome (HIV-1) reverse transcriptase such as AZT, d4T, ddI, 3TC and ddC which are chain terminating nucleoside analogs. We investigated atomic charges, regioselective patterns of chemical activity and other indices of biochemical activity in order to obtain a better understanding of how the drugs work and the mechanism of drug resistance. HF and DFT methods were used including diffusion, polarization and correlation effects to obtain fully optimized geometric parameters. We investigated the effects of solvents, Mulliken and natural bond orbital charge distributions, vibrational frequencies and hydrogen bond effects [2].

In 2004 we reported computer-aided molecular design of novel glucosidase inhibitors for AIDS treatment. One of the targets is the glucosidase protein, which depends on the activity of enzymes such as glucosidase and transferase for the elaboration of the polysaccharides. The DFT method was used to investigate several glucosidase inhibitors and ligand/receptor interactions. Analysis of the interactions of the proposed pharmaceutical (a pseudodisaccharide, with the Thermotoga maritime 4-alpha-glucanotransferase in complex with modified acarbose), the scores from docking as well as the superposition of all the ligands, suggest that our molecular designed pseudo-dissacharide may be a potent glucosidase inhibitor [3].

In 2004 we also reported a molecular modeling and QSAR study of suppressors of the growth of Trypanasoma cruzi epimastigotes. We studied 18 dithiocarbamate suppressors of the growth of Trypanosoma cruzi epimastigotes reported in the literature as superoxide dismutase (SOD) inhibitors. Principal component analysis indicated that the descriptors, heat of formation, logarithm of the partition coefficient, superficial area, charge of the nitrogen atom from the ditiocarbamate group as well as charges from the two carbon atoms adjacent to nitrogen are responsible for the classification between the lower and higher trypanomacid activity. Using docking methods and multiple linear regression methods it was possible to identify the probable bioactive isomers that suppress the growth of T. cruzi epimastiotes. Our best partial least square (PLS) model obtained with the descriptors yields a good correlation between experimental and predicted biological activities. Quantum chemical semi-empirical AM1 and PM3 calculations were performed for the lowest energy conformations of the compounds as well as other topological and three-dimensional molecular descriptors with the purpose of representing different sources of chemical information in terms of molecular size, shape, symmetry and atom distribution in the molecule [4].

In 2004 we also published the work density functional and docking studies of retinoids for cancer treatment. The retinoic acid receptor (RAR) and retinoid X receptor (RXR) are members of the nuclear receptor superfamily. The ligand-binding domain contains the ligand-dependent activation function. The isotypes RAR α β γ are distinct pharmacological targets for retinoids involved in the treatment of various cancers and skin diseases. There is thus considerable interest in synthetic retinoids with isotype selectivity and reduced side effects. The retinoid acid receptors and three of its panagonists were investigated. We carried out DFT as well as the electrostatic potential calculations. Docking was used to study the interactions between the receptor and the three ligands. We proposed a theoretically more potent inhibitor, which can be obtained by modifying one of the retinoic acids investigated [5].

In 2005 we published a work on molecular dynamics, database screening, density functional and docking studies of novel RAR ligands in cancer chemotherapy [6, 528].

We also published in 2005 our results regarding a rational design of novel diketoacid-containing ferrocene inhibitors of HIV-1 integrase [7].

In 2005 we reported our research on computer-aided design of a novel ligand for retinoic acid receptor in cancer chemotherapy [8].

We also published in 2005 a paper on homology modeling and molecular interaction field studies of α-glicosidases as a guide to structure-based design of novel proposed anti-HIV inhibitors [9].

In 2006 we reported the ADMET properties, database screening, molecular dynamics, density functional and docking studies of novel potential anti-cancer compounds. Quantum chemical calculations were performed to obtain partial charges, and docking of molecules using large databases. We optimized ~350,000 molecules at the AM1 level in order to obtain geometries and charges for docking calculations. Promising new ligands were optimized by DFT. From the molecular trajectory of the systems generated by the molecular dynamics simulations we analyzed the root mean square-deviation of each system with respect to all atoms as well as the trial energy as function of time. The absorption, distribution, metabolism, excretion and toxicity properties as well as the parameters of the Rule of Five were investigated. Comparisons were made with a crystallographic ligand of RAR. Our novel proposed anti-cancer ligand indicates hydrophobic and strong polar interactions with the receptor [10].

In 2006 we also published the book Modern Biotechnology in Medicinal Chemistry and Industry [11].

In 2006 we also reported a molecular dynamics, docking, density functional and ADMET studies of HIV-1 reverse transcriptase inhibitors. Nucleoside analogs constitute a family of biological molecules (ddI, d4T, ddC and 3TC) which play an important role in the transcription process of the human immunodeficiency virus. The normal nucleoside substrates used by reverse transcriptase (RT) to synthetize DNA are mimicked by these nucleoside analogs that lacked a 3'-OH group and consequently act as chain terminators when incorporated in the DNA by RT. We performed molecular dynamics, density functional with correlation as well as docking of inhibitors of HIV-1 reverse transcriptase RT. The objective was to propose a novel potential HIV-1 RT inhibitor RTI, which introduces new hydrogen bond interactions and has high docking scores. The molecular dynamics studies, analysis of the ligand-receptor interactions in the active site as well as ADMET properties suggests advantages for this potential RTI [12].

In 2007 we reported computer-aided molecular design of novel HMG-CoA reductase inhibitors for the treatment of hyhpercholesterolemia [532]. Elevated cholesterol levels are a primary risk factor for the development of coronary artery disease. HMG-CoA reductase is an important molecular target of hypolipemic drugs, known as statins, which are effective in the reduction of cholesterol serum levels. We used density functional theory, flexible docking, molecular dynamics as well as ADMET and synthetic accessibility analyses in order to propose novel potential HMG-CoA reductase inhibitors. These are designed by bioiososeric modification and are promising for the treatment of hypercholesterolemia [13].

We also reported in 2007 virtual screening, molecular interaction fields molecular dynamics with explicit water solvation, docking, density functional and ADMET properties of novel AChE inhibitors in Alzheimer's disease (AD). This disease is characterized by senile plaquets and cholinergic deficits. Many drugs currently used for the treatment of AD are based on the improvement of cholinergic neurotransmission achieved by Acetylcholinestarase (AChE) inhibition, the enzyme responsible for acetylcholine hydrolysis. The complexes of AChE with inhibitors were computer-aided designed by us. Toxicity and Metabolism predictions, flexible docking as well as MIF studies were also made. Using the various models discussed above we proposed novel potential AChE inhibitors for the treatment of Alzheimer's disease [14].

In 2007 we published the first volume of our Enciclopedia: Current Methods in Medicinal Chemistry and Biological Physics [15].

In 2008 we performed molecular dynamics, flexible docking, virtual screening, ADMET predictions and molecular interaction fields studies to design novel potential MAO-B inhibitors which act on well-known targets for antidepressant, Parkinson's disease and neuroprotecive drugs. We performed optimizations, flexible docking and virtual screening in large databases. Toxicity predictions were performed and the 'Rule of Five' (RO5) was calculated for these proposals. We thus designed new molecules with potential higher selectivity and enzymatic inhibitory activity over MAO-B [16].

In 2008 we also reported molecular dynamics, density functional, ADMET predictions, virtual screening, molecular interaction field studies for identification and evaluation of novel potential CDK2 (cyclin-dependent kinases responsible for the progression of cells through the various phases and transitions of the cell cycle) inhibitors in cancer therapy. Eight novel potential inhibitors of CDK2 were proposed showing interesting structural characteristics that are required for inhibiting the CDK2 activity indicating potential as drug candidates for CDK2-based cancer therapy [17].

We also investigated in 2008 virtual screening, flexible docking and molecular interaction fields to design novel HMG-CoA reductase inhibitors for the treatment of hyhpercholesterolemia [18].

In 2008 we investigated pharmacokinetic and pharmacodynamic predictions of novel potential HIV-1 integrase inhibitors [19].

In 2008 we published the second volume of our Enciclopedia: Current Methods in Medicinal Chemistry and Biological Physics [20].

In 2008 we also published an Invited Mini Review on Current Topics in Computer-aided Drug Design [21].

In 2009 we reported computer-aided drug design of novel Phospholipase A_2 (PLA$_2$) inhibitor candidates for treatment of snakebites. We did the PLA$_2$ BthTX-I structure prediction based on homology modeling as well as a virtual screening in a large database yielding a set of potential bioactive inhibitors. Molecular interaction fields indicated important binding effects. We proposed a theoretically nontoxic, drug-like, and potential novel BthTX-1 inhibitor. Our calculations were used to design novel phospholipase inhibitors for future treatment of snakebite victims as well as other human diseases in which PLA$_2$ enzymes are involved [22, 540].

In 2010 we reported computer-aided drug design and ADMET predictions for identification and evaluation of novel potential farnesyltransferase inhibitors in cancer therapy [541]. Ras protein is a cell component that controls growth and multiplication whereas an abnormal form of the signaling Ras is present in almost 30% of cancers. Methods capable of neutralizing Ras are useful in the fight against cancer. We used molecular dynamics, density functional theory, virtual screening, ADMET predictions and molecular interaction field studies to design, analyze and propose novel potential inhibitors of Farnesyltransferase. Some proposals indicate theoretically interesting pharmacotherapeutic profiles, when compared to the very active and most cited FTase inhibitors. This yields alternative scaffolds to design future potential FTase inhibitors in the fight against cancer [23].

In 2010 we published our book Recent Developments in Medicinal Chemistry, 2010, Vol 1 [24].

We reported in 2010 our invited contribution stoichiometry of amino acids driven protein folding? [25].

In 2011 we reported a simple, practical, and efficient protocol for drug design, in particular diabetes, which includes selection of the illness, good choice of a target as well as a bioactive ligand, and then usage of various computer aided drug design and medicinal chemistry tools to design novel potential drug candidates in different diseases. We selected the validated target dipeptidyl peptidase IV (DPP-IV), whose inhibition contributes to reduce glucose levels in type 2 diabetes patients. The most active inhibitors were extracted from the BindingDB database. By using including flexible docking, virtual screening, molecular. interaction fields, molecular dynamics, ADME, and toxicity predictions we proposed 4 novel potential DDP-IV inhibitors with drug properties for Diabetes control [26].

In 2011 we reported work on homology modeling, virtual screening and molecular dynamics of the MARK3 KA1 domain for cancer drug design. Structural homology modeling was done with the software AMPS, MODELLER, PROCHECK, WHATIF AND VERIFY-3D to generate a quality model of human MARK3. Virtual screening identifies the principal residues of MARK3 which interact with the ligands. The pharmacophoric model obtained from Discovery Studio coincides with those obtained by molecular interaction fields. Our investigations using virtual screening with pharmacophoric constraints as well as molecular dynamics indicates the most stable compounds in the ligand sitel. Also indicated is their potential toxicities yielding inhibitors for further investigations of human MARK3 KA1 domain with potential for the treatment of head and neck cancer [27].

In 2011 we investigated *in silico* design and search for acetylcholinerase inhibitors in Alzheimer's disease with a suitable pharmacokinetic profile and low toxicity. Alzheimer"s disease is a complex neurodegenerative disorder of the central nervous system, characterized by amyloid-$\beta\beta$ deposits, $\tau\tau$-protein aggregation, oxidative stress and reduced levels of acetylcholine in the brain.

One pharmacological approach is to restore acetylcholine level by inhibiting acetylcholinesterase (AChE) with reversible inhibitors, such as galanthamine. We investigated AChE-drug complexes (1QT1 and 1ACJ PDB codes making ligand-binding sites calculations within the active site of the enzyme, pharmacophore perception of galanthamine derivatives, virtual screening, toxicophorical analysis and estimation of pharmacokinetics properties. Four galanthamine derivatives having a N-alkyl-Ph chain were designed; In addition 12 drug-like compounds from the Ilibdiverse database were selected by virtual screening as novel, hypothetical AChE inhibitors. The molecules have the potential to guide the design of drugs with optimized pharmacodynamic and pharmacokinetic properties in order to improve the treatment of Alzheimer"s disease (new pharmacotherapeutic options) [28].

In 2011 we published a paper on toxicophoric and metabolic *in silico* evaluation of benzimidazole and phenylbenzamide derivatives with potential application as anticancer agents. Absorption, distribution, metabolism, excretion and toxicity information, *in silico* predictions are an interesting alternative to evaluate prototypes during early stages of the drug design processes. Benzimidazole and a phenylbenzamide derivatives, previously identified as novel anticancer lead compounds (which can prevent DNA binding to hnRNP K protein) were evaluated *in silico* regarding their metabolic profile and toxicity potential. Phenylbenzamide derivative seems to be a molecule with better pharmaceutical profile, since the possible metabolites present a milder degree of chemical structure toxic alerts. For the benzimidazole derivative one possible strategy would be to replace the benzimidazole ring system by bioisosteres with lower toxic potential [29].

In 2012 we published our book chapter An overview of tropical parasitic diseases: Causative agents, targets and drugs [30].

In 2013 we published the paper 'Comments on the paper Levinthal's question, revisited, and answered [31].

In 2013 we published our mini-review on Phospolipase A2 inhibitors isolated from medicinal plants: Alternative treatments against snakebites [32].

In 2013 we reported studies of targets for inhibition of proinflamatory cytokines linked to CNS disorders in preclinical animal models, including Alzheimer's diseases, lateral sclerosis, cerebral ischemia and neurophatic pain. We made similarity-based and pharmacophore virtual screening of approximately 18.3

million compounds. Our research was based on a correlation between the specific binding mode and activity of different types of p38α MAPK inhibitors. Novel potential inhibitors were proposed [33].

We also reported in 2013 structure and ligand based rational drug design for Bace-1 inhibitors We designed novel inhibitors of BACE-1 starting from structures available in the Protein Data Bank and performing virtual screening of libraries, evaluation of toxicity prediction, pharmacokinetic properties and analysis of binding modes in the catalytic site [34].

In 2013 we published our work on density Functional Theory, Molecular Interaction Fields, Pharmacophore, Virtual Screening and Physical Chemistry of the Interactions of Novel Acetylcholinesterase Inhibitors in Alzheimer's Disease. The research on acetylcholinesterase (AChE) has increased due to discoveries indicating the involvement of the enzyme in the formation of the β-amiloid peptide during the pathogenesis of Alzheimer's disease.

It has been noted that this enzyme plays a key role in acceleration of the senile plaques of β-amiloid peptide which is toxic for the neurons. For the development of new potential inhibitors of the enzyme AChE, different techniques of molecular modeling were used as a strategy for the rational design of pharmaceuticals. The basis was the AChE inhibitors described in the literature in addition to those deposited in the PDB and commercial compounds with properties of pharmaceuticals [35].

In 2014 we published pharmacophore-based drug design of novel potential Tau ligands for Alzheimer's disease treatment. In this work we use selected pharmacophoric model to perform pharmacophore-based virtual screening in order to design novel potential Tau aggregation inhibitors. Prediction of biological activity and pharmaceutical properties indicated promising Tau aggregation inhibitors for Alzheimer's treatment [36].

In 2014 we also published molecular dynamics, density functional theory, pharmacophoe modeling, molecular interaction fields, pharmacodynamic, pharmacokinetic toxicity investigation of novel bioactive compounds interacting with CDK2 surfaces. We have proposed novel potential CDK2 inhibitors as well as molecular modifications of known inhibitors and evaluated them with respect to pharmacodynamic and pharmacokinetic-toxicity properties [37].

ACKOWLEDGEMENTS

We acknowledge financial support from CNPQ, FAPERJ, FAPESP.

CONFLICTS OF INTEREST

The author confirms that this chatper contents have no conflict of itnerest.

REFERENCES

[1]   Martins JBL, Perez MA, Silva CHTP, Taft CA, Arissawa M, Longo E, Mello PC, Stamato FMLG and Tostes JGR. Theoretical *ab initio* study of ranitidine. International Journal of Quantum Chemistry. 2002, 90:575-586.

[2]   Arissawa M, Taft CA, Felcman J. Investigation of nucleoside analogs with anti-HIV activity. International Journal of quantum chemistry 2003, 93:422-432.

[3]   Silva CHTP and Taft CA. Computer-aided molecular design of novel glucosidase inhibitors for AIDS treatment. Journal of biomolecular structure and dynamics. 2004, 22:59-63.

[4]   Silva CHTP, Sanches SM and Taft CA. A molecular modeling and QSAR study of suppressors of the growth of Trypanasoma cruzi espimastigotes. J. Mol. Graph and Modeling 2004, 3:89-97.

[5]   Silva CHTP, Almeida P, Taft CA. Density functional and docking studies of retinoids for cancer treatment. J. Mol. Model 2004,10:38-43.

[6]   Silva CHTP and Taft CA. Molecular dynamics, database screening, density functional and docking studies of novel RAR ligands in cancer chemotherapy 2005, 117:73-77.

[7]   Silva CHTP, Del Ponte G, Neto AF, Taft CA. Rational design of novel diketoacid-containing ferrocene inhibitors of HIV-1 integrase. Bioorganic Chemistry. 2005,33:274-284.

[8]   Silva CHTP, Leopoldino AM, Silva EHT, Espinoza VAA and Taft CA. Computer-aided design of a novel ligand for retinoic acid receptor in cancer chemotherapy. Int. J. of Quantum. Chem. 2005, 102:1131-1135.

[9]   Silva CHTP, Carvalho I and Taft CA. Homology modeling and molecular interaction Field studies of α-glucosidases as a guide to structure-based design of novel proposed anti-HIV inhibitors. J. of Computer-Aided Molecular Design. 2005, 1983-92.

[10]   Silva CHTP and Taft CA. ADMET properties, database screening, Molecular dynamics, density functional and docking studies of novel potential anti-cancer compounds. J. of Biomolecular structure & dynamics.2006;24,263-268.

[11]   Modern biotechnology in medicinal chemistry and industry; 2006; Editor: Carlton A. Taft, Research Signpost, Kerala, India.

[12]   Silva CHTP and Carvalho I. Molecular dynamics, docking, density functional and ADMET studies of HIV-1 reverse transcriptase inhibitors. J. of Theoretical and Computationa Chemistry 2006,5:579-586.

[13]   da Silva VB, Andrioli WJ, Carvalho I, Taft CA and Silva CHTP. Computer-aided molecular design of novel HMG-CoA reductase inhibitors for the treatment of hypercholesterolemia. J. Theor. and Comput. Chem. 2007, 6:811-821.

[14]   Silva CHTP, Carvalho I and Taft CA. Virtual screening, molecular interaction field, molecular dynamics docking, density functional and ADMET properties of novel AchE inhibitors in Alzheimer's disease. J. of Biomolecular Structure & Dynamics. 2007, 24:515-523.

[15]   Current Methods in Medicinal Chemistry and Biological Physics. 2007, Vol. 1, Editors Carlton A. Taft and Carlos H. T. P. Silva, 2007, Research Signpost, Kerala, India

[16]   Braun GH, Jorge DMM, Ramos HP, Alves RM, Guilliati S, Sampaio SV, Taft and Silva CHTP. Molecular dynamics, flexible docking, virtual screening. ADMET predictions and molecular interaction field studies to design novel potential MAO-B inhibitors. J. of Biomolecular structure & dynamics 2008, 25:347-355.

[17]   da Silva VB, Kawano DF, Gomes AS, Carvalho I, Taft CA, Silva CHTP. Molecular dynamics, density functional, ADMET predictions, virtual screening and molecular interaction Field studies for identification and evaluation of novel potential CDK2 inhibitors in cancer therapy. J. Phys. Chem. A 2008, 112:8902-8910.

[18]   Silva CHTP, DA Silva VB and Taft CA. Use of virtual screening, flexible docking and molecular interaction fields to design novel HMG-CoA reductase inhibitors for the treatment of hypercholesterolemia. J. Phys. Chem. A 2008, 112:2007-2011.

[19]   Silva CHTP, da Silva VB and Taft CA. Pharmacokinetic and pharmacodynamic predictions of novel potential HIV-1 integrase inhibitors. Drug metabolism letters 2008, 2:256-260.

[20]   Current Methods in Medicinal Chemistry and Biological Physics. 2008, Vol. 2. Editors Carlton A. Taft and Carlos H. T. P. Silva, Research Signpost, Kerala, India.

[21]   Taft CA, Silva CHTP, Invited Mini Review: Current Topics in Computer-aided Drug Design, Journal of Pharmaceutical Sciences, 2008, 97: 89-1098

[22]   Hage-Mellim LIS, Silva CHTP, Semighini EP, Taft CA and Sampaio SV. Computer-aided drug design of novel PLA$_2$ inhibitor candidates for treatment of snakebite. J. of Biomolecular Structure & dynamics 2009, 27:27-36.

[23]   Silva CHTP, da Silva VB, Resende J, Rodrigues PF, Bononi FC, Benevenuto CG and Taft CA, Computer-aided drug design and ADMET predictions for identification and evaluation of novel potential farnesyltransferase inhibitors in cancer therapy J. of Molecular Graphics and Modeling. 2010, 28:513-523.

[24]   Recent developments in Medicinal Chemistry, 2010, Editors: Carlton A. Taft and Carlos H. T. P. Silva, Bentham Science Publishers (UAE).

[25]   Silva CHTP, Taft CA. Stoichiometry of amino acids drives protein folding? Journal of Biomolecular Structure & Dynamics, 2010, 28:635- 636.

[26]   Semighini EP, Resende J, Andrade P, Morais PAB, Carvalho I, Taft CA, Silva CHTP. Using Computer-aided Drug Design and Medicinal Chemistry Strategies in the Fight Against Diabetes. Journal of Biomolecular Structure & Dynamics, 2011, 28: 787-796, 2011.

[27]   Semighini EP, Taft CA, Silva CHTP, Homology modeling, virtual screening and molecular dynamics of the MARK3 KA1 domain for cancer drug design. Molecular Simulation, 2011, 37:1199-1219.

[28] Taft CA, da Silva VB, de Andrade P, Kawano DF, Morais PAB, Almeida JR, Carvalho I, Taft CA and Silva CHTP. *In silico* design and search for acetylcholinesterase inhibitors in Alzheimer's disease with a suitable pharmacokinetic profile and low toxicity, Future Medicinal Chemistry, 2011, 3: 947- 960.

[29] da Silva VB, Leopoldino AM, Silva CHTP, Taft CA, Toxicophoric and Metabolic *In Silico* Evaluation of Benzimidazole and Phenylbenzamide Derivatives with Potential Application as Anticancer Agents. Drug Metabolism Letters, 2011, 5:267- 275.

[30] Taft CA and Silva CHTP. An Overview of Tropical Parasitic Diseases: Causative Agents, Targets and Drugs. In Chemoinformatics: Directions Toward Combating Neglected Diseases. Bentham Sci. Pub. (Dubai, U.A.E.) Eds. T. C. Ramalho, M. P. Freitas and E. F. F. da Cunha. 2012. Pp. 174-196.

[31] Taft CA. Silva CHTP, Silva CHTP, Comments on the paper Levinthals question, revisited, and answered, Journal of Biomolecular Structure & Dynamics. 2013,13:1001-1002.

[32] Hage-Melim L, Sampaio S, Taft CA, Silva CHTP, Phospholipase A2 Inhibitors Isolated From Medicinal Plants: Alternative Treatment Against Snakebites. Mini-Reviews in Medical Chemistry, 2013, 13: 1348-1356.

[33] Pinsetta FR, Taft CA, Silva CHTP, Rational Design of Novel Potential p38α MAPK Inhibitors with Drug-like Properties using pharmacophore and Similarity-based Virtual Screening Procedures. Current Bioactive Compounds. 2013, 13: 3-13.

[34] Semighini EP, Taft CA, Silva CHTP, Structure and Ligand Based Rational Drug Design for Bace-1 Inhibitors. Current Bioactive Compounds, 2013, 9: 14-20.

[35] Almeida JR, Taft CA, Silva CHTP. Density Functional Theory, Molecular Interaction Fields, Pharmacophore, Virtual Screening and Physical Chemistry of the Interactions of Novel Acetylcholinesterase Inhibitors in Alzheimer's Disease. Current Physical Chemistry. 2013, 3: 419-430.

[36] Susimaire Pedersoli-Mantoani, Vinicius Barreto da Silva, Carlton Anthony Taft and Carlos Henrique Tomich de Paula da Silva. Pharmacophore-based Design of Novel Potential Tau Ligands for Alzheimer's Disease Treatment, Current Physical Chemistry, 2014, 4:35-44.

[37] Ferreira FP, Couto WF, Fontana F, Taft CA, da Silva CHTP. Molecular Dynamics, Density Functional Theory, Pharmacophore Modeling, Molecular Interaction Fields, Pharmacodynamic, Pharmacokinetic Toxicity Investigation of Novel Bioactive Compounds Interacting with CDK2 Surfaces. Current Physical Chemistry, 2014, 4:94-105.

[38] Paul SM, Mytelka DS, Dunwiddlie CT, Persinger CC, Munon BH, Lindorbg SR, Schacht AL How to improve R&D roducivity; the pharmaceutical industry's grand challenge. Nat Rev Drug Discov. 2010, 9:203-214.

[39] Stouch TR, The errors of our ways: taking account of error in computer-aided drug design to build confidence intervals for our next 25 years, J. Comput. Aided Mol. Des. 2012, 26:125-134.

[40] Dongyue C, Junmei W, Rui Z, Youyong L, Huidong Y and Tingjun H. Evaluation in Drug Discovery. PharmacoKinetics Knowledge Base (PKKB):A Comprehensive Database of Pharmacokinetic and Toxic Properties for Drugs, J. Chem. Inf. Model., 2012, 52: 1132-1134

[41] Greer J, Erickson JW, Baldwin JJ, Varney MD, Application of the three-dimensional structures of protein target molecules in structure-based drug design. J. Med. Chem. 1994, 37:1035-1054.

[42]   Gund P, Wipke WT, Langridge R Computer searching of a molecular structure file for pharmacophoric patterns. Comput Chem Res Educ Technol, 1974, 3:5-21

[43]   Martin YC, Bures MG, Willett P (1990) Searching databases of three-dimensional structures. In: Lipkowitz K, Boyd D (eds) Reviews in computational chemistry, vol 1. VCH, Weinheim, pp 213-263

[44]   Sheridan RP, Venkataraghavan R. Designing novel nicotinic agonists by searching a database of molecular shapes. J Comput Aided Mol Des 1987,1:243-256

[45]   Lewis RA, Dean PM. Automated site-directed drug design: the formation of molecular templates in primary structure generation.Proc R Soc Lond B, 1989, 236:141-162

[46]   VanDrie JH, Weininger D, Martin YC. ALADDIN: an integrated tool for computer-assisted molecular design and pharmacophore recognition from geometric, steric, and substructure searching of three-dimensional molecular structures. J Comput Aided Mol Des 1989, 3:225-240

[47]   Bartlett PA, Shea GT, Telfer SJ, Waterman S. CAVEAT: a program to facilitate the structure-derived design of biologically active molecules. In: Roberts SM (ed) Molecular recognition in chemical and biological problems, vol 78. Spec Publ R Soc Chem, Cambridge. 1989, pp 182-196

[48]   Lauri G, Bartlett PA. CAVEAT: a program to facilitate the design of organic molecules. J Comput Aided Mol Des. 1994, 8:51-66

[49]   Carhart RE, Smith DH, Gray NAB, Nourse JG, Djerassi C. GENOA: a computer program for structure elucidation utilizing overlapping and alternative substructures. J Org Chem. 1981, 46: 1708-1718.

[50]   Wise M, Cramer RD, Smith D, Exman I. Progress in three- dimensional drug design: the use of real time color graphics and computer postulation of bioactive molecules in DYLOMMS.In:Dearden JC (ed) Quantitative approaches to drug design. Elsevier, Amsterdam, 1983. pp 145-146

[51]   Goodford PJ. A computational procedure for determining energetically favorable binding sites on biologically important macromolecules. J Med Chem. 1995, 28:849-857

[52]   Nishibata Y, Itai A. Automatic creation of drug candidate structures based on receptor structure. Starting point for artificial lead generation. Tetrahedron 1991, 47:8985-8990

[53]   Nishibata Y, Itai A. Confirmation of usefulness of a structure construction program based on three-dimensional receptor structure for rational lead generation. J Med Chem. 1993, 36: 2921-2928

[54]   Bohm HJ. The computer program LUDI: a new method for the *de novo* design of enzyme inhibitors. J Comput Aided Mol Des. 1992, 6:61-78

[55]   Bohm HJ. LUDI: rule-based automatic design of new substituents for enzyme inhibitor leads. J Comput Aided Mol Des, 1992, 6:593-606

[56]   Loving K, Alberts I, Sherman W. Computational approaches for fragment-based and *de novo* design. Curr Top Med Chem. 2010, 10:14-32

[57]   Hartenfeller M, Schneider G. Enabling future drug discovery by *de novo* design. WIREs Comp Mol Sci. 2011, 1:742-759

[58]   Schneider G, Fechner U. Computer-based *de novo* design of drug-like molecules. Nat Rev Drug Discov. 2005, 4:649-663

[59]   Reutlinger M, Guba W, Martin RE, Alanine AI, Hoffmann T, Klenner A, Hiss JA, Schneider P, Schneider G. Neighborhood-preserving visualization of adaptive structure-

activity landscapes:Application to drug discovery. Angew Chem Int Ed Engl. 2011, 50: 11633-11636.

[60] Schneider G, Hartenfeller M, Reutlinger M, Tanrikulu Y, Proschak E, Schneider P. Voyages to the unknown: adaptive design of bioactive compounds.Trends Biotechnol. 2009, 27:18-26

[61] Miranker A, Karplus M. Functionality maps of binding sites: a multiple copy simultaneous search method. Proteins. 1991, 11: 29-34

[62] Kuntz ID, Blaney JM, Oatley SJ, Langridge R, Ferrin TE. A geometric approach to macromolecule-ligand interactions. J Mol Biol. 1982, 161:269-288

[63] Cramer RD, Patterson DE, Bunce JD. Comparative molecular field analysis (CoMFA). 1. Effect of shape on binding of steroids to carrier proteins. J Am Chem Soc.1988, 110:5959-5967

[64] Jackson RC. Update on computer-aided drug design. Curr Opin Biotechnol. 1995, 6:646-651

[65] Bo-Lm HJ (1996) Current computational tools for *de novo* ligand design. Curr Opin Biotechnol. 1996, 7:433-436

[66] Bohacek RS, McMartin C. Modern computational chemistry and drug discovery: structure generating programs. Curr Opin Chem Biol. 1997, 1:157-161

[67] Marrone TJ, Briggs JM, McCammon JA. Structure-based drug design: computational advances. Annu Rev Pharmacol Toxicol. 1997, 37:71-90

[68] Kubinyi H. Combinatorial and computational approaches in structure-based drug design. Curr Opin Drug Discov Devel. 1998, 1:16-27

[69] Moon JB, Howe WJ. Computer design of bioactive molecules: a method for receptor-based *de novo* ligand design. Proteins. 1991, 11:314-328

[70] Bohacek RS, McMartin C. Multiple highly diverse structures complementary to enzyme binding sites: results of extensive application of a *de novo* design method incorporating combinatorial growth. J Am Chem Soc. 1994, 116:5560-5571

[71] Schneider G, Neidhart W, Giller T, Schmid G. 'Scaffold hopping' by topological pharmacophore search: a contribution to virtual screening. Angew Chem Int Ed Engl. 1999, 38:2894-2896

[72] Alig L, Alsenz J, Andjelkovic M, Bendels S, Benardeau A, Bleicher K, Bourson A, David-Pierson P, Guba W, Hildbrand S, Kube D, Lubbers T, Mayweg AV, Narquizian R, Neidhart W, Nettekoven M, Plancher JM, Rocha C, Rogers-Evans M, RO ver S, Schneider G, Taylor S, Waldmeier P. Benzodioxoles: novel cannabinoid-1 receptor inverse agonists for the treatment of obesity. J Med Chem. 2008, 51:2115-2127

[73] Mauser HG. Recent developments in *de novo* design and scaffold hopping. Curr Opin Drug Discov Devel. 2010, 11:365-374

[74] Langdon SR, Ertl P, Brown N. Bioisosteric replacement and scaffold hopping in lead generation and optimization. Mol Inf. 2010, 29:366-385

[75] Bailey D, Brown D. High-throughput chemistry and structure-based design: survival of the smartest. Drug Discov Today. 2001, 6:57-59

[76] Bleicher KH, Bo HM, Muller K, Alanine AI. Hit and lead generation: beyond high-throughput screening. Nat Rev Drug Discov, 2003, 2:369-378

[77] Schneider G. Virtual screening: an endless staircase? Nat Rev Drug Discov. 2010, 9:273-276

[78] Kruger BA, Dietrich A, Baringhaus KH, Schneider G. Scaffold-hopping potential of fragment-based *de novo* design: the chances and limits of variation. Comb Chem High Throughput Screen. 2009, 12: 383-396

[79] Heridan RP, Rusinko A III, Nilakantan R, Venkataraghavan R. Searching for pharmacophores in large coordinate data bases and its use in drug design. Proc Natl Acad Sci USA. 1989, 86:8165-8169

[80] Babine RE, Bleckman TM, Kissinger CR, Showalter R, Pelletier Beddell CR, Goodford PJ, Norrington FE, Wilkinson S, Wootton R. Compounds designed to fit a site of known structure in human haemoglobin. Br J Pharmacol. 1976, 57:201-209

[81] Beddell CR, Goodford PJ, Norrington EE, Wilkinson S and Wootton R. Compounds designed to fit on site of human haemoglobin. Br J. Pharmacol. 1979, 57:207-209.

[82] Lewell XQ, Judd DB, Watson SP, Hann MM. RECAP-retrosynthetic combinatorial analysis procedure: a powerful new technique for identifying privileged molecular fragments with useful applications in combinatorial chemistry. J Chem Inf Comput Sci. 1998, 38:511-522.

[83] Vinkers HM, de Jonge MR, Daeyaert FF, Heeres J, Koymans LM, van Lenthe JH, Lewi PJ, Timmerman H, Van Aken K, Janssen PA. SYNOPSIS: synthesize and optimize system *in silico*. J Med Chem. 2003, 46:2765-2773

[84] Schneider G, Lee ML, Stahl M, Schneider P. *De novo* design of molecular architectures by evolutionary assembly of drug-derived building blocks. J Comput Aided Mol Des. 2000, 14: 487-494

[85] Wang R, Gao Y, Lai L. LigBuilder: a multi-purpose program for structure-based drug design. J Mol Model, 2000, 6:498-516

[86] Kandil S, Biondaro S, Vlachakis D, Cummins AC, Coluccia A, Berry C, Leyssen P, Neyts J, Brancale A. Discovery of a novel HCV helicase inhibitor by a *de novo* drug design approach, 2009,19: 2935-2937.

[87] Feher M, Gao Y, Baber JC, Shirley WA, Saunders J. The use of ligand-based *de novo* design for scaffold hopping and sidechain optimization: two case studies. Bioorg Med Chem. 2008, 16:422-427

[88] Lanier MC, Feher M, Ashweek NJ, Loweth CJ, Rueter JK, Slee DH, Williams JP, Zhu YF, Sullivan SK, Brown MS. Selection, synthesis, and structure-activity relationship of tetrahydropyrido[4, 3-d]pyrimidine-2, 4-diones as human GnRH receptor antagonists. Bioorg Med Chem. 2007, 15:5590-5603.

[89] Rogers-Evans M, Alanine A, Bleicher K, Kube D, Schneider G (2004) Identification of novel cannabinoid receptor ligands *via* evolutionary *de novo* design and rapid parallel synthesis. QSAR Comb Sci. 2004, 26:426-430

[90] Schneider G, Designing the molecular future, J. Comput. Aided Mol. Des. 2012, 26:115-120.

[91] Cavasotto CN, Homology models in docking and high-throughput docking, Current Topics in Medicinal Chemistry, 2011, 11: 1528-1554.

[92] Cavasotto, CN, Orry AJ. Ligand docking and structure-based virtual screening in drug discovery. Curr. Top. Med. Chem., 2007, 7: 1006-1014.

[93] Levitt M. Growth of novel protein structural data. Proc. Natl. Acad. Sci. USA, 2007, 104: 3183-3188.

[94] Lundstrom K. Structural genomics and drug discovery. J. Cell Mol. Med., 2007, 11: 224-238.

[95]   Manjasetty BA, Turnbull AP, Panjikar S, Bussow K, Chance MR. Automated technologies and novel techniques to accelerate protein crystallography for structural genomics Proteomics, 2008, 8: 612-625.

96]   Mooij WT, Hartshorn MJ, Tickle IJ, Sharff AJ, Verdonk ML,Jhoti H. Automated protein-ligand crystallography for structure-based drug design. Chem Med Chem, 2006, 1: 827-838.

[97]   Alkhalfioui F, Magnin T, Wagner R, From purified GPCRs to drug discovery: the promise of protein-based methodologies. Curr. Opin. Pharmacol. 2009, 9: 629-635.

[98]   Pieper U, Eswar N, Webb BM, Eramian D, Kelly L, Bar- Kan DT, Carter H, Mankoo P, Karchin R, Marti-Renom MA, Davis FP, Sali A. MODBASE, a database of annotated comparative protein structure models and associated resources. Nucleic Acids Res., 2009, 37: D347-D354.

[99]   Tuccinardi T. Docking-based virtual screening: recent developments. Comb. Chem. High Throughput Screen, 2009, 12: 303-314.

[100]   Cavasotto CN, Phatak, S. S. Homology modeling in drug discovery: current trends and applications. Drug Discov. Today, 2009, 14: 676-683.

[101]   Hillisch A, Pineda LF, Hilgenfeld R. Utility of homology models in the drug discovery process. Drug Discov. Today, 2004, 9: 659-669.

[102]   Costanzi S, On the applicability of GPCR homology models to computer-aided drug discovery:a comparison between *in silico* and crystal structures of the beta2-adrenergic receptor. J. Med. Chem., 2008, 51: 2907-2914.

[103]   Phatak SS, Gatica EA, Cavasotto CN. Ligand-steered modeling and docking: A benchmarking study in class A G-protein-coupled receptors. J. Chem. Inf. Model., 2010, 50: 2119-2128.

[104]   Michino M, Abola E, Brooks CL, Dixon JS, Moult J, Stevens RC. Community-wide assessment of GPCR structure modeling and ligand docking: GPCR Dock 2008. Nat. Rev. Drug Discov. 2009, 8: 455-463.

[105]   Cavasotto CN, Orry AJ, Murgolo NJ, Czarniecki MF, Kocsi SA, Hawes BE, O'Neill KA, Hine H, Burton MS, Voigt JH, Abagyan RA, Bayne ML. Monsma FJ Jr. Discovery of novel chemotypes to a G-protein-coupled receptor through ligand-steered homology modeling and structure-based virtual screening Med.Chem. 2008, 1: 581-588.

[106]   Altschul SF, Madden TL, Schaffer AA, Zhang J, Zhang Z, Miller W, Lipman DJ. Gapped BLAST and PSI-BLAST: a new generation of protein database search programs. Nucleic Acids Res, 1997, 25: 3389-3402.

[107]   Edgar RC, Sjolander KA. comparison of scoring functions for protein sequence profile alignment. Bioinformatics, 2004, 20: 1301-1308.

[108]   Krogh A, Brown M, Mian IS, Sjolander K, Haussler D. Hidden Markov models in computational biology. Applications to protein modeling. J. Mol. Biol., 1994, 235:1501-1531.

[109]   Cheng J. A multi-template combination algorithm for protein comparative modeling. BMC Struct. Biol., 2008, 8: 8-18.

[110]   Jamroz M, Kolinski A. Modeling of loops in proteins: a multimethod approach. BMC Struct.Biol. 2011, 10: 5-10.

[111]   Villoutreix BO. Eudes R, Miteva MA. Structure-based virtual ligand screening: recent success stories. Comb. Chem. High Throughput Screen, 2009, 12: 1000-1016.

112]   Cavasotto CN, Phatak SS. Docking methods for structure- based library design. Methods Mol. Biol., 2011, 685: 155-174.

[113]   Amaro RE, Li WW. Emerging methods for ensemble-based virtual screening. Curr. Top. Med. Chem., 2010, 10: 3-13.

[114]   Cavasotto CN. Normal mode-based approaches in receptor ensemble docking. Methods Mol. Biol. 2011, 2011, 51: 1604-1622.

[115]   Cavasotto CN, Singh N. Docking and high throughput docking: successes and the challenge of protein flexibility. Curr. Comput.Aided Drug Des., 2008, 4: 221-234.

[116]   Spyrakis F, Bidon-Chanal, A, Barril X, Luque FJ. Protein flexibility and ligand recognition: challenges for molecular modeling. Curr. Top. Med. Chem, 2011, 11: 192-210

[117]   Cozzini P, Kellogg GE, Spyrakis F, Abraham DJ, Costantino G, Emerson A, Fanelli F, Gohlke H, Kuhn LA. Morris, Morris GM, Orozco M, Pertinhez TA, Rizzi M, Sotriffer CA. Target flexibility: an emerging consideration in drug discovery and design. J Med Chem. 2008,51: 6237-6255.

[118]   Orozco M, Pertinhez TA, Rizzi M, Sotriffer CA. Target flexibility: an emerging consideration in drug discovery and design. J. Med. Chem., 2008, 51: 6237-6255.

[119]   Barillari C, Taylor J, Viner R, Essex JW. Classification of water molecules in protein binding sites. J. Am. Chem. Soc., 2007, 129: 2577-2587.

[120]   Marti-Renom MA, Stuart AC, Fiser A, Sanchez R, Melo F, Sali A. Comparative protein structure modeling of genes and genomes. Annu. Rev. Biophys. Biomol. Struct., 2000, 29: 291-325.

[121]   Canutescu AA, Shelenkov AA, Dunbrack RL Jr. A graphtheory algorithm for rapid protein side-chain prediction. Protein Sci., 2003, 12: 2001-2014.

[122]   Dunbrack RL, Karplus M. Backbone-dependent rotamer library for proteins. Application to side-chain prediction. J. Mol. Biol., 1993, 230: 543-574.

[123]   Sali A, Blundell TL. Comparative protein modeling by satisfaction of spatial restraints. J. Mol. Biol. 1993, 234: 779-815.

[124]   Evers A, Klebe G. Ligand-supported homology modeling of g-protein-coupled receptor sites: models sufficient for successful virtual screening. Angew. Chem. Int Ed. Engl., 2004, 43: 248-251.

[125]   Evers A, Klebe G. Successful virtual screening for a submicromolar antagonist of the neurokinin-1 receptor based on a ligand-supported homology model. J. Med. Chem., 2004, 47: 5381-5392.

[126]   Moro S, Deflorian F, Bacilieri M, Spalluto G. Ligand-based homology modeling as attractive tool to inspect GPCR structural plasticity. Curr. Pharm. Des., 2006, 12: 2175-2185.

[127]   Sherman W, Day T, Jacobson MP, Friesner RA, Farid R. Novel procedure for modeling ligand/receptor induced fit effects. J. Med. Chem., 2006, 49: 534-553.

[128]   Orry AJW, Cavasotto CN. In: Ligand-docking-based homology model of the Melanin-Concentrating Hormone 1 receptor, 231st Meeting of the American Chemical Society, Atlanta, GA, 2006; Atlanta, GA, 2006.

[129]   Diaz P, Phatak SS, Xu J, Astruc-Diaz F, Cavasotto CN, Naguib M. 6-Methoxy-N-alkyl isatin acylhydrazone derivatives as a novel series of potent selective cannabinoid receptor 2 inverse agonists: Design, synthesis and binding mode prediction. J. Med. Chem., 2009, 52: 433-444.

[130] Diaz P, Phatak SS, Xu J, Fronczek FR, Astruc-Diaz F. Thompson CM, Cavasotto CN, Naguib M. 2,3-Dihydro-1- benzofuran derivatives as a series of potent selective cannabinoid receptor 2 agonists: design, synthesis, and binding mode prediction through ligand-steered modeling. Chem Med Chem, 2009, 4: 1615-1629.

[131] Lin MS, Head-Gordon T. Reliable protein structure refinement using a physical energy function. J. Comput. Chem., 2011, 32: 709-717.

[132] Cavasotto CN, Kovacs JA, Abagyan RA. Representing Receptor Flexibility in Ligand Docking through Relevant Normal Modes. J. Am. Chem. Soc., 2005, 127: 9632-9640.

[133] Kovacs JA, Cavasotto CN, Abagyan RA. Conformational Sampling of Protein Flexibility in Generalized Coordinates: Application to ligand docking. J. Comp. Theor. Nanosci, 2005, 2: 354- 361.

[134] Rai BK, Tawa GJ, Katz AH. Humblet C. Modeling G protein-coupled receptors for structure-based drug discovery using low-frequency normal modes for refinement of homology models: application to H3 antagonists. Proteins, 2010, 78: 457-473.

[135] Sperandio O, Mouawad L, Pinto E, Villoutreix BO, Perahia D, Miteva MA. How to choose relevant multiple receptor conformations for virtual screening: a test case of CDK2 and normal mode analysis. Eur. Biophys. J., 2010, 39: 1365-1372.

[136] Cavasotto CN, Abagyan RA. Protein flexibility in ligand dock-ing and virtual screening to protein kinases. J. Mol. Biol., 2004, 337: 209-225.

[137] Cavasotto CN, Liu G, James SY, Hobbs PD, Peterson VJ, Bhattacharya AA, Kolluri S K, Zhang XK, Leid M, Abagyan R, Liddington RC, Dawson MI. Determinants of retinoid X receptor transcriptional antagonism. J. Med. Chem., 2004, 47: 4360-4372.

[138] Monti MC, Casapullo A, Cavasotto CN, Napolitano A, Riccio R. Scalaradial, a dialdehyde-containing marine metabolite that causes an unexpected noncovalent PLa(2) inactivation. ChemBioChem, 2007, 8: 1585-1591.

[139] Monti MC, Casapullo A, Cavasotto CN, Tosco A, Dal Piaz F, Ziemys A, Margarucci L, Riccio R. The binding mode of petrosaspongiolide M to the human group IIA phospholipase A(2): exploring the role of covalent and noncovalent interactions in the inhibition process. Chem.-Eur. J. 2009, 15: 1155-1163.

[140] Vilar S, Ferino G, Phatak SS, Berk B, Cavasotto CN, Costanzi S. Docking-based virtual screening for GPCRs ligands: not only crystal structures but also *in silico* models. J. Mol. Graph. Model. 2011, 29: 614-623.

[141] Fan H, Schneidman-Duhovny D, Irwin JJ, Dong G, Schoichet BK, Sali A, Statistical potential for modeling and ranking of protein-ligand interactions, J. Chem. Inf. Mol, 2011, 51: 3078-3092.

[142] Garcia-Sosa AT, Hetenyi C, Maran U, Drug efficiency indices for improvement of molecular docking scoring functions, J. Comput. Chem, 2011,31: 174-184.

[143] Bordogna A, Pandini A, Bonati L, Predicting the accuracy of protein-ligand docking on homology models, J. Comput. Chem. 2011, 32: 81-98.

[144] Obiol-Pardo, Lopez L, Pastor M, Selent J, Progress in the structural prediction of G protein-coupled receptors:D_3 receptor in complex with eticlopride, Proteins, 2011, 79:1695-17703.

[145] Phatak SS, Gatica EA, Cavasotto CN, Ligand-steered modeling and docking a benchmarking study in class a G-protein-coupled receptors, J. Chem. Inf. Model, 2010, 50:2119-2128.

[146} McRobb FM, Capuano B, Crosby IT, Chalmers D, Yuriev E, Homology modeling and docking evaluation of aminergic G protein-coupled receptors, j. Chem. Inf. Model, 2010, 50:626-637.

[147] de Graaf C, Kooistra AJ, Vischer HF, Katritch V, Kujer M, Shiroishi M, Iwata S, Shimamura T, Stevens RC, de Esch U, Leurs R, Crysal structure-based virtual screening for fragment-like ligands of the human histamine H(1) receptor, J. Med. Chem, 2011, 54:8195-8206.

[148] Hsieh JH, YinS, Liu S, Sedyakh A, Dokholyan NV, Tropsha A, Combined application of chemoinformatics-and physical force field-based scoring functions improves binding affinity prediction for CSAR data sets, J. Chem. Inf. Models, 2011, 51:2027-2035.

[149] Tang H, Wang XS, Hsieh JH, Tropsha A. Do crystal structures obviate the need for theoretical models of GPCRs for structure-based virtual screening? Proteins, 2012:30: 1503-1521.

[150] Sheng C and Zhang W, Computational fragment-based drug design:An overview and update, Medicinal Research Reviews, 2013, 33:554-598.

[151] Verdonk ML, Giangreco I, Hall Rj, Korb O, Mortenson PN, Murray CW, 2011, Docking performance of fragments and drug like compounds, J. Med. Chem. 2011, 54:5422-5431.

[152] Villar HO, Hansen MR. Computational techniques in fragment based drug discovery. Curr Top Med Chem 2007,7:1509-1513.

[153] Zoete V, Grosdidier A, Michielin O. Docking, virtual high throughput screening and *in silico*, fragment-based drug design. J Cell Mol Med 2009,13:238-248.

[154] Makara GM. On sampling of fragment space. J Med Chem 2007, 50:3214-3221.

[155] Faller B, Ertl P. Computational approaches to determine drug solubility. Adv Drug Deliv Rev 2007, 59:533-545.

[156] Fejzo J, Lepre CA, Peng JW, Bemis GW, Ajay, Murcko MA, Moore JM. The SHAPES strategy: An NMR-based approach for lead generation in drug discovery. Chem Biol 1999, 6:755-769.

[157] Lepre C. Fragment-based drug discovery using the SHAPES method. Expert Opin Drug Discov 2007, 2:1555-1566.

[158] Chung S, Parker JB, Bianchet M, Amzel LM, Stivers JT. Impact of linker strain and flexibility in the design of a fragment-based inhibitor. Nat Chem Biol, 2009,5:407-413.

[159] Schneider G, Fechner U. Computer-based *de novo* design of drug-like molecules. Nat Rev Drug Discov 2005, 4:649-663.

[160] Zhu Z, Sun ZY, Ye Y, Voigt J, Strickland C, Smith EM, Cumming J, Wang L, Wong J, Wang YS, Wyss DF, Chen X, Kuvelkar R, Kennedy ME, Favreau L, Parker E, McKittrick BA, Stamford A, Czarniecki M, Greenlee W, Hunter JC. Discovery of cyclic acylguanidines as highly potent and selective beta-site amyloid cleaving enzyme (BACE) inhibitors: Part I-Inhibitor design and validation. J Med Chem, 2010,53:951-965.

[161] Johnson MC, Hu Q, Lingardo L, Ferre RA, Greasley S, Yan J, Kath J, Chen P, Ermolieff J, Alton G. Novel isoquinolone PDK1 inhibitors discovered through fragment-based lead discovery. J Comput Aided Mol Des 2011, 25:689-698.

[162] Congreve M, Carr R, Murray C, Jhoti H. A 'rule of three' for fragment-based lead discovery? Drug Discov Today 2003, 8:876-877.

[163] Card GL, Blasdel L, England BP, Zhang C, Suzuki Y, Gillette S, Fong D, Ibrahim PN, Artis DR, Bollag G, Milburn MV, Kim SH, Schlessinger J, Zhang KY. A family of

phosphodiesterase inhibitors discovered by co-crystallography and scaffold-based drug design. Nat Biotechnol 2005, 23:201-207.

[164] Davies DR, Mamat B, Magnusson OT, Christensen J, HaraldssonMH, Mishra R, Pease B, Hansen E, Singh J, Zembower D, Kim H, Kiselyov AS, Burgin AB, Gurney ME, Stewart LJ. Discovery of leukotriene A4 hydrolase inhibitors using metabolomics biased fragment crystallography. J Med Chem 2009, 52:4694-4715.

[165] Law RJ. Tetrabromobisphenol A: Investigating the worst-case scenario. Mar Pollut Bull 2009, 58:459-460.

[166] Bondensgaard K, Ankersen M, Thogersen H, Hansen BS, Wulff BS, Bywater RP. Recognition of privileged structures by G-protein coupled receptors. J Med Chem 2004,47:888-899.

[167] Schnur DM, Hermsmeier MA, Tebben AJ. Are target-family-privileged substructures truly privileged? J Med Chem 2006, 49:2000-2009.

[168] Clark M, Wiseman JS. Fragment-based prediction of the clinical occurrence of long QT syndrome and torsade de pointes. J Chem Inf Model 2009, 49:2617-2626.

[169] Oprea TI, Blaney JM. Cheminformatics approaches to fragment-based lead discovery. In: Jahnke W, Erlanson DA, Eds. Fragment-Based Approaches in Drug Discovery. Methods and Principles in Medicinal Chemistry, Vol. 34. Weinheim: Wiley-VCH Verlag GmbH, 2006. pp 91-111.

[170] Tanaka N, Ohno K, Niimi T,Moritomo A, Mori K, OritaM. Small-world phenomena in chemical library networks: Application to fragment-based drug discovery. J Chem Inf Model 2009, 49:2677-2686.

[171] Chen H, Gao J, Lu Y, Kou G, Zhang H, Fan L, Sun Z, Guo Y, Zhong Y. Preparation and characterization of PE38KDEL-loaded anti-HER2 nanoparticles for targeted cancer therapy.J Control Release 2008,128:209-216.

[172] Lewell XQ, Judd DB, Watson SP, Hann MM. RECAP—Retrosynthetic combinatorial analysis procedure: A powerful new technique for identifying privileged molecular fragments with useful applications in combinatorial chemistry. J Chem Inf Comput Sci. 1998, 38:511-522.

[173] Parn J, Degen J, Rarey M. Exploring fragment spaces under multiple physicochemical constraints. J Comput Aided Mol Des 2007,21:327-340.

[174] Durrant JD, Amaro RE, McCammon JA. AutoGrow: A novel algorithm for protein inhibitor design. Chem Biol Drug Des 2009, 73:168-178.

[175] Morris GM, Goodsell DS, Halliday RS, Huey R, Hart WE, Belew RK, Olson AJ. Automated docking using a Lamarckian genetic algorithm and an empirical binding free energy function. J Comput Chem 1998, 19:1639-1662.

[176] Kutchukian PS, Lou D, Shakhnovich EI. FOG: Fragment Optimized Growth algorithm for the *de novo* generation of molecules occupying drug-like chemical space. J Chem Inf Model 2009,49:1630-1642.

[177] Pearlman DA, Murcko MA. CONCERTS: Dynamic connection of fragments as an approach to *de novo* ligand design. J Med Chem. 1996,39:1651-1663.

[178] Bohm HJ. The computer program LUDI:A new method for the *de novo* design of enzyme inhibitors. J Comput Aided Mol Des 1992,6:61-78.

[179] Bohm HJ. On the use of LUDI to search the Fine Chemicals Directory for ligands of proteins of known three-dimensional structure. J Comput Aided Mol Des 1994,8:623-632.

[180] Lauri G, Bartlett PA. CAVEAT: A program to facilitate the design of organic molecules. J Comput Aided Mol Des 1994, 8:51-66.

[181] Tschinke V, Cohen NC. The NEWLEAD program: A new method for the design of candidate structures from pharmacophoric hypotheses. J Med Chem. 1993,36:3863-3870.

[182] Miranker A, Karplus M. An automated method for dynamic ligand design. Proteins 1995,23:472-490.

[183] Stahl M, Todorov NP, James T, Mauser H, Boehm HJ, Dean PM. A validation study on the practical use of automated *de novo* design. J Comput Aided Mol Des 2002, 16:459-478.

[184] Dey F, Caflisch A. Fragment-based *de novo* ligand design by multiobjective evolutionary optimization. J Chem Inf Model 2008, 48:679-690.

[185] Majeux N, Scarsi M, Apostolakis J, Ehrhardt C, Caflisch A. Exhaustive docking of molecular fragments with electrostatic solvation. Proteins 1999, 7:88-105.

[186] Ji H, Stanton BZ, Igarashi J, Li H, Martasek P, Roman LJ, Poulos TL, Silverman RB. Minimal pharmacophoric elements and fragment hopping, an approach directed at molecular diversity and isozyme selectivity. Design of selective neuronal nitric oxide synthase inhibitors. J Am Chem Soc 2008, 130:3900-3914.

[187] Ji H, Li H, Martasek P, Roman LJ, Poulos TL, Silverman RB. Discovery of highly potent and selective inhibitors of neuronal nitric oxide synthase by fragment hopping. JMedChem 2009, 52:779-797.

[188] Yuan Y, Pei J, Lai L. LigBuilder 2: A practical *de novo* drug design approach. J Chem Inf Model 2011, 51:1083-1091.

[189] Wang R, Gao Y, Lai L. A multi-purpose program for structure-based drug design. J Mol Model 2000, 6:498-516.

[190] Boda K, Seidel T, Gasteiger J. Structure and reaction based evaluation of synthetic accessibility. J Comput Aided Mol Des 2007, 21:311-325.

[191] Meunier B. Hybrid molecules with a dual mode of action: Dream or reality? Acc Chem Res 2008, 41:69-77.

[192] Viegas-Junior C, Danuello A, da Silva Bolzani V, Barreiro EJ, Fraga CA.Molecular hybridization: A useful tool in the design of new drug prototypes. Curr Med Chem 2007, 14:1829-1852.

[193] Pierce AC, Rao G, Bemis GW. BREED: Generating novel inhibitors through hybridization of known ligands. Application to CDK2, p38, and HIV protease. J Med Chem 2004, 47:2768-2775.

[194] Li Y, Zhao Y, Liu Z, Wang R. Automatic tailoring and transplanting: A practical method that makes virtual screening more useful. J Chem Inf Model. 2011,51:1474-1491.

[195] Nisius B, Rester U. Fragment shuffling: An automated workflow for three-dimensional fragmentbased ligand design. J Chem Inf Model. 2009, 49:1211-1222.

[196] Moriaud F, Doppelt-Azeroual O, Martin L, Oguievetskaia K, Koch K, Vorotyntsev A, Adcock SA, Delfaud F. Computational fragment-based approach at PDB scale by protein local similarity. J Chem Inf Model. 2009, 49:280-294.

[197] Doppelt O, Moriaud F, Bornot A, de Brevern AG. Functional annotation strategy for protein structures. Bioinformation 2007,1:357-359.

[198] Jambon M, Andrieu O, Combet C, Deleage G, Delfaud F, Geourjon C. The SuMo server: 3D search for protein functional sites. Bioinformatics 2005, 21:3929-3930.

[199] Schneider G, Neidhart W, Giller T, Schmid G. "Scaffold-Hopping" by topological pharmacophore search: A contribution to virtual screening. Angew Chem Int Ed Engl 1999, 38:2894-2896.

[200] Baringhaus KH, Hessler G. Fast similarity searching and screening hit analysis. Drug Discovery Today, Technol 2004, 1:197-204.

[201] Maass P, Schulz-Gasch T, Stahl M, Rarey M. Recore: A fast and versatile method for scaffold hopping based on small molecule crystal structure conformations. J Chem Inf Model 2007, 47:390-399.

[202] Schneider G, Hartenfeller M, Reutlinger M, Tanrikulu Y, Proschak E, Schneider P. Voyages to the (un)known: Adaptive design of bioactive compounds. Trends Biotechnol 2009, 27:18-26.

[203] Hajduk PJ, Greer J. A decade of fragment-based drug design: Strategic advances and lessons learned. Nat Rev Drug Discov. 2007, 6:211-219.

[204] Shuker SB, Hajduk PJ, Meadows RP, Fesik SW. Discovering high-affinity ligands for proteins: SAR by NMR. Science 1996, 274:1531-1534.

[205] Chessari G, Woodhead AJ. From fragment to clinical candidate—A historical perspective. Drug Discov Today 2009, 14:668-675.

[206] Schuffenhauer A, Ruedisser S, Marzinzik AL, Jahnke W, Blommers M, Selzer P, Jacoby E. Library design for fragment based screening. Curr Top Med Chem 2005, 5:751-762.

[207] Siegal G, Ab E, Schultz J. Integration of fragment screening and library design. Drug Discov Today 2007, 12:1032-1039.

[208] Lepre CA, Moore JM, Peng JW. Theory and applications of NMR-based screening in pharmaceutical research. Chem Rev 2004, 104:3641-3676.

[209] Swayze EE, Jefferson EA, Sannes-Lowery KA, Blyn LB, Risen LM, Arakawa S, Osgood SA, Hofstadler SA, Griffey RH. SAR byMS: A ligand based technique for drug lead discovery against structured RNA targets. J Med Chem 2002, 45:3816-3819.

[210] Erlanson DA, Wells JA, Braisted AC. Tethering:Fragment-based drug discovery. AnnuRev Biophys Biomol Struct 2004, 33:199-223.

[211] Hartshorn MJ, Murray CW, Cleasby A, Frederickson M, Tickle IJ, Jhoti H. Fragment-based lead discovery using X-ray crystallography. J Med Chem 2005, 48:403-413.

[212] Danielson UH. Fragment library screening and lead characterization using SPR biosensors. Curr Top Med Chem 2009, 9:1725-1735.

[213] Neumann T, Junker HD, Schmidt K, Sekul R. SPR-based fragment screening: Advantages and applications. Curr Top Med Chem 2007, 7:1630-1642.

[214] Rees DC, Congreve M, Murray CW, Carr R. Fragment-based lead discovery. Nat Rev Drug Discov 2004, 3:660-672.

[215] Flaherty KT, Yasothan U, Kirkpatrick P. Vemurafenib. Nat Rev Drug Discov 2011,10:811-812.

[216] Murray CW, Rees DC. The rise of fragment-based drug discovery. Nat Chem 2009, 1:187-192.

[217] Congreve M, Chessari G, Tisi D, Woodhead AJ. Recent developments in fragment-based drug discovery. J Med Chem 2008,51:3661-3680.

[218] Zartler ER, Shapiro MJ. Fragonomics: Fragment-based drug discovery. Curr Opin Chem Biol 2005, 9:366-370.

[219] Bembenek SD, Tounge BA, Reynolds CH. Ligand efficiency and fragment-based drug discovery. Drug Discov Today 2009, 14:278-283.

[220] Fruh V, Zhou Y, Chen D, Loch C, Ab E, Grinkova YN, Verheij H, Sligar SG, Bushweller JH, Siegal G. Application of fragment-based drug discovery to membrane proteins:

Identification of ligands of the integral membrane enzyme DsbB. Chem Biol 2010, 17:881-891.

[221]   Bamborough P, Brown MJ, Christopher JA, Chung CW, Mellor GW. Selectivity of kinase inhibitor fragments. J Med Chem 2011, 54:5131-5143.

[222]   Babaoglu K, Shoichet BK. Deconstructing fragment-based inhibitor discovery. Nat Chem Biol 2006,2:720-723.

[223]   Warr WA. Fragment-based drug discovery: What really works. An interview with Sandy Farmer of Boehringer Ingelheim. J Comput Aided Mol Des 2011,25:599-605.

[224]   Desjarlais RL. Using computational techniques in fragment-based drug discovery. Methods Enzymol 2011, 493:137-155.

[225]   Gozalbes R, Carbajo RJ, Pineda-Lucena A. Contributions of computational chemistry and biophysical techniques to fragment-based drug discovery. Curr Med Chem 2010,17:1769-1794.

[226]   Hoffer L, Renaud JP, Horvath D. Fragment-based drug design: Computational & experimental state of the art. Comb Chem High Throughput Screen 2011, 14:500-520.

[227]   Hubbard RE, Chen I, Davis B. Informatics and modeling challenges in fragment-based drug discovery.Curr Opin Drug Discov Devel 2007,10:289-297.

[228]   Law R, Barker O, Barker JJ, Hesterkamp T, Godemann R, Andersen O, Fryatt T, Courtney S, Hallett D, Whittaker M. The multiple roles of computational chemistry in fragment-based drug design. J Comput Aided Mol Des 2009,23:459-473.

[229]   Vangrevelinghe E, Rudisser S. Computational approaches for fragment optimization. Curr Comput-Aided Drug Design 2007, 3:69-83.

[230]   Houston DR and Walkinshaw MD, Consensus Docking:Improving the reliability of ocking in a virtual screening context, J. Chem. Inf. And Modeling, 2013,53: 384-290.

[231]   Badrinarayan P, Sastry GN, Virtual high throughput screening in new lead identification. Comb. Chem. High throughput Screeen. 2011,14:840-860.

[232]   Langdon SR, Ertl P and Brown N, Bioisosteric replacement and scaffold hopping in lead generation and optimization, Mol. Inf. 2010, 29: 366-385.

[233]   Devereux M and Popelier PLA, *In silico* techniques for the identification of bioisosteric replacements for drug design, Current Topics in medicinal chemistry, 2010, 10: 657- 668.

[234]   Devereux M, Popelier PLA, McLay IM. Toward an *Ab initio* fragment database for bioisosterism: dependence of QCT properties on level of theory, conformation, and chemical environment. J. Comp. Chem., 2009, 30: 1300-1318.

[235]   Devereux M, Popelier PA, McLay IM. A refined model for prediction of hydrogen bond acidity and basicity parameters from quantum chemical molecular descriptors. Phys.Chem. Chem. Phys., 2009, 11: 1595-1603.

[236]   Wagener M. Lommerse JPM. The quest for bioisosteric replacements. J. Chem. Inf. Model., 2006, 46: 677-685.

[237]   Toropov AA, Toropova AP, Benfenati E, Leszczynska D, Leszczynski J. SMILES-based optimal descriptors: QSAR analysis of fullerene-based HIV-1 PR inhibitors by means of balance of correlations. J. Comp. Chem., 2010, 31: 381-92.

[238]   Karelson M, Lobanov VS, Katritzky AR. Quantum-chemical descriptors in QSAR/QSPR studies. Chem. Rev., 1996, 96: 1027-1043.

[239]   Kortagere S, Krasowski MD and Ekins S. The importance of discerning shape in molecular pharmacology. Trends in Pharmacological Sciences. 2009,30:138-147

[240] Popelier PLA, Smith PJ. QSAR models based on quantum topological molecular similarity. Eur. J. Med. Chem., 2006, 41: 862-873.

[241] Lamarche O, Platts JA, Hersey A. Theoretical prediction of partition coefficients *via* molecular electrostatic and electronic properties. J. Chem. Inf. Comput. Sci., 2004, 44: 848-855.

[242] Kennewell EA, Willett P,Ducrot P, Luttmann C. Identification of target-specific bioisosteric fragments from ligand protein crystallographic data. J. Comput. Aided Mol. Des., 2006, 20: 385-394.

[243] Nicholls A, MacCuish NE, MacCuish JD. Variable selection and model validation of 2D and 3D molecular descriptors. J. Comp. Aided Mol. Des., 2004, 18: 451-474

[244] Sidhu PS, Mosier PD, Zhou Q, Desai UR, On scaffold hopping: Challenges in the discovery of sulfated small molecules as mimetics of glycosaminoglycans, Bioorganic & Medicinal Chemistry Letters. 2013, 23: 355-359.

[245] ZhaoH, Scaffold selection and scaffold hopping in lead generation: a medicinal chemistry perspective, Drug Discovery Today, 2007, 12: 149-155.

[246] Sun H, Tawa G and Wallqvist A, Classification of scaffold hopping approaches, Drug Discovery Today, 2012, 17: 310-324.

[247] Brown N and Jacoby E, On scaffolds and hopping in medicinal chemistry. Mini Rev. Med. Chem. 2006, 6: 1217-1229

[248] Mauser H and Guba W. Recent developments in *de novo* design and scaffold hopping. Curr. Opin. Drug Discov. Dev. 2008, 11: 365-374

[249] Renner S, and Schneider GSm Scaffold-hopping potential of ligand-based similarity concepts. ChemMedChem. 2006, 1: 181-185

[250] Zhang Q. and Muegge I. Scaffold hopping through virtual screening using 2D and 3D similarity descriptors: ranking, voting, and consensus scoring. J. Med. Chem. 2006, 49: 1536-1548

[251] Wassermann AM and Bajorath J. Chemical substitutions that introduce activity cliffs across different compound classes and biological targets. J. Chem. Inf. Model, 2010, 50: 1248-1256.

[252] Brown N and Jacoby E, On scaffolds and hopping in medicinal Chemistry, Mini-Reviews in Medicinal Chemistry, 2006, 6:1217-1220.

[253] Mauser H and Guba W. Recent developments in *de novo* design and scaffold hopping. Curr. Opin. Drug Discov. Dev. 2008, 11: 365-374

[254] Wassermann AM and Bajorath J, Chemical substitutions that introduce activity cliffs across different compound classes and biological targets. J. Chem. Inf. Model. 2010, 50: 1248-1256

[255] Yang SY, Pharmacophore modeling and applications in drug discovery: challenges and recent advances. Drug Discov. Today. 2010, 15: 444-450.

[256] Jerez JM, Jerez M, Garcia CG, Ballester S, Castro A, Combined use of pharmacophoric models together with drug metabolism and genotoxicity *in silico* studies in the hit finding process, J. Comput. Aided Mol. Des., 2013, 27:79-90.

[257] Dong X, Ebalunode JO, Yang SY, and Zheng W, Receptor-Based Pharmacophore and Pharmacophore Key Descriptors for Virtual Screening and QSAR Modeling Current Computer-Aided Drug Design, 2011, 7: 181-189

[258] Van Drie JH. Monty Kier and the origin of the pharmacophore concept. Internet Electron. J. Mol. Des., 2007, 6: 271-279.

[259]   Kier LB. Molecular orbital calculation of preferred conformations of acetylcholine, muscarine, and muscarone. Mol. Pharmacol.1967, 3: 487-494.

[260]   Barnum D, Greene J, Smellie A, Sprague P, Identification of common functional configurations among molecules. J. Chem. Inf. Comput. Sci., 1996, 36: 563-571.

[261]   Jones G, Willett P, Glen RC, A genetic algorithm for flexible molecular overlay and pharmacophore elucidation. J. Comput. Aided Mol. Des., 1995, 9: 532-549.

[262]   Richmond NJ, Abrams CA, Wolohan PR, Abrahamian E, Willett P, Clark RD, GALAHAD: Pharmacophore identification by hypermolecular alignment of ligands in 3D. J.Comput. Aided Mol. Des. 2006, 20: 567-587.

[263]   Dixon SL, Smondyrev AM, Knoll EH, Rao SN, Shaw DE, Friesner RA,PHASE: a new engine for pharmacophore perception, 3D QSAR model development, and 3D database screening: 1. Methodology and preliminary results. J. Comput. Aided Mol. Des., 2006, 20: 647-671.

[264]   Dixon SL, Smondyrev AM, Rao SN, PHASE: a novel approach to pharmacophore modeling and 3D database searching. Chem. Biol. Drug Des., 2006, 67: 370-372.

[265]   Bandyopadhyay D, Agrafiotis DK, A self-organizing algorithm for molecular alignment and pharmacophore development. J. Comput. Chem., 2008, 29: 965-982.

[266]   Feng J. Sanil A, Young SS. PharmID: pharmacophore identification using Gibbs sampling. J. Chem. Inf. Model., 2006, 46: 1352-1359.

[267]   Jones G. GAPE: an improved genetic algorithm for pharmacophore elucidation. J. Chem. Inf. Model., 2010, 50: 2001-2018.

[268]   Langer T, Pharmacophores in drug research. Mol. Inf., 2010, 29:470-475.

[269]   Sanders MPA, McGuire R, Roumen L, de Esch IJP, de Vlieg J, Klompe JPG and de Graaf C. From the protein's perspective: the benefits and challenges of protein structure-based pharmacophore modeling. Med. Chem. Commun., 2012, 3: 28-38

[270]   Sotriffer CA, Accounting for induced-fit effects in docking: What is possible and what is not?, Current Topics in Medicinal Chemistry, 2011, 11:179-191.

[271]   May A, Sieker, F, Zacharias, M. How to efficiently include receptor flexibility during computational docking. Curr. Comput. Aided Drug Des., 2008, 4: 143-153.

[272]   Wong CF, Flexible ligand-flexible protein docking in protein kinase systems. Biochim. Biophys. Acta, 2008, 1784: 244-251.

[273]   B-Rao, C, Subramanian, J, Sharma SD. Managing protein flexibility in docking and its applications. Drug Discov. Today, 2009, 14: 394-400.

[274]   Henzler AM, Rarey M, Protein flexibility in structure-basevirtual screening: from models to algorithms. In: Virtual Screening Sotriffer C., Ed.; Wiley VCH: Weinheim, 2011.

[275]   Jiang F, Kim, SH. "Soft docking": matching of molecular surface cubes. J. Mol. Biol., 1991, 219: 79-102.

[276]   Kokh DB, Wenzel W, Flexible side chain models improve enrichment rates in *in silico* screening. J. Med. Chem., 2008, 51:5919-5931.

[277]   Gschwend DA, Good AC, Kuntz ID. Molecular docking towards drug discovery. J. Mol. Recognit., 1996, 9: 175-186.

[278]   Leach AR. Ligand docking to proteins with discrete side-chain flexibility. J. Mol. Biol., 1994, 235: 345-356.

[279]   Schaffer L. Verkhivker GM, Predicting structural effects iHIV-1 protease mutant complexes with flexible ligand docking and protein side-chain optimization. Proteins: Struct., Funct., Bioinform., 1998, 33: 295-310.

[280] Schnecke V, Swanson CA, Getzoff ED, Tainer JA, Kuhn LA. Screening a peptidyl database for potential ligands to proteins with side-chain flexibility. Proteins: Struct., Funct., Bioinf., 1998,33: 74-87.

[281] Jones G, Willett P. Glen RC. Molecular recognition of receptosites using a genetic algorithm with a description of desolvation. Mol. Biol., 1995, 245: 43-53.

[282] Frauenfelder H, Sligar SG, Wolynes PG. The energy landscapes and motions of proteins. Science, 1991, 254: 1598-1603.

[283] Teague SJ. Implications of protein flexibility for drug discovery. Nat. Rev. Drug Discov., 2003, 2: 527-541.

[284] Ahmed A, Kazemi S, Gohlke H, Protein flexibility and mobility in structure-based drug design. Front. Drug Des. Discov. 2007, 3: 455-476.

[285] Cozzini P, Kellogg GE, Spyrakis, F, Abraham, DJ, Costantino G, Emerson A, Fanelli F, Gohlke H, Kuhn LA, Morris GM, Orozco M, Pertinhez TA.; Rizzi M, Sotriffer CA. Target flexibility: an emerging consideration in drug discovery and design. J. Med. Chem., 2008, 51: 6237-6255.

[286] MacRaild CA, Daranas AH, Bronowska A, Homans SW. Global changes in local protein dynamics reduce the entropic cost of carbohydrate binding in the arabinose-binding protein. J. Mol. Biol., 2007, 368: 822-832.

[287] Perola E, Charifson PS. Conformational analysis of drug-like molecules bound to proteins: an extensive study of ligand reorganization upon binding. J. Med. Chem., 2004, 47: 2499-2510.

[288] Gutteridge A, Thornton J. Conformational changes observed in enzyme crystal structures upon substrate binding. J. Mol. Biol., 2005, 346: 21-28.

[289] Najmanovich R, Kuttner J, Sobolev V, Edelman M. Side-chain flexibility in proteins upon ligand binding. Proteins: Struct., Funct. Bioinform., 2000, 39: 261-268.

[290] Mobley DL, Dill KA. Binding of small-molecule ligands to proteins: "what you see" is not always "what you get". Structure, 2009, 17: 489-498.

[291] Koshland DE. Application of a theory of enzyme specificity to protein synthesis. Proc. Natl. Acad. Sci. USA, 1958, 44: 98-104.

[292] Rarey M, Kramer B, Lengauer T, Klebe G. A fast flexible docking method using an incremental construction algorithm. J.Mol. Biol., 1996, 261: 470-489.

[293] Rarey M, Kramer B, Lengauer T. Multiple automatic base selection: protein-ligand docking based on incremental construction without anual intervention. J. Comput. Aided Mol. Des., 1997, 11: 369-384.

[294] Ewing TJ, Makino S, Skillman AG, Kuntz ID. DOCK 4.0: search strategies for automated molecular docking of flexible molecule databases. J. Comput. Aided Mol. Des., 2001, 15: 411-428.

[295] Warren GL, Andrews C W, Capelli AM, Clarke B, LaLonde J, Lambert MH,. Lindvall M, Nevins N, Semus SF, Senger S, Tedesco G, Wall ID, Woolven JM, Peishoff CE, Head MS. A critical assessment of docking programs and scoring functions. J. Med. Chem., 2006, 49: 5912-5931.

[296] Abagyan R, Totrov M. High-throughput docking for lead generation. Curr. Opin. Chem. Biol., 2001, 5: 375-382.

[297] Carlson HA, McCammon JA. Accommodating protein flexibility in computational drug design. Mol. Pharmacol., 2000, 57: 213-218.

[298] Carlson HA. Protein flexibility and drug design: how to hit a moving target. Curr. Opin. Chem. Biol., 2002, 6: 447-452.

[299] Teodoro ML, Kavraki LE. Conformational flexibility models for the receptor in structure based drug design. Curr. Pharm. Des., 2003, 9:1635-1648.

[300] Cavasotto CN, Orry AJW, Abagyan RA. The challenge of considering receptor flexibility in ligand docking and virtual screening. Curr. Comput. Aided Drug Des., 2005, 1: 423-440.

[301] Totrov M. Abagyan R. Flexible ligand docking to multiple receptor conformations: a practical alternative. Curr. Opin. Struct. Biol., 2008, 18: 178-184.

[302] Muegge, I. Rarey, M. Small molecule docking and scoring. In: Reviews in Computational Chemistry, Lipkowitz, K.B., Boyed, D.B. Eds. Wiley-VCH: New York, 2001; vol. 17, pp. 1-60.

[303] Halperin I, Ma B, Wolfson H, Nussinov R. Principles of docking: An overview of search algorithms and a guide to scoring functions. Proteins: Struct., Funct., Bioinform., 2002, 47: 409-443.

[304] Sotriffer CA, Stahl M, Boehm HJ, Klebe G. Docking and Scoring Functions / Virtual Screening. In: Burger's Medicinal Chemistry and Drug Discovery, 6th ed., D. J. Abraham, ED.; Wiley: New York, 2003; Vol. 1, pp. 281-333.

[305] Brooijmans N, Kuntz ID. Molecular recognition and docking algorithms. Annu. Rev. Biophys. Biomol. Struct., 2003, 32: 335-373.

[306] Sousa SF, Fernandes PA, Ramos MJ. Protein-ligand docking: current status and future challenges. Proteins: Struct., Funct. Bioinf., 2006, 65: 15-26.

[307] Moitessier N, Englebienne P, Lee D, Lawandi J, Corbeil CR. Towards the development of universal, fast and highly accurate docking/scoring methods: a long way to go. Br. J. Pharmacol. 2008, 153: S7-S26.

[308] Davis IW, Baker D. RosettaLigand docking with full ligand and receptor flexibility. J. Mol. Biol., 2009, 385: 381-392.

[309] Schnecke V, Kuhn LA. Virtual screening with solvation and ligand-induced complementarity. Perspect. Drug Discov. Des. 2000, 20: 171-190.

[310] Abagyan R, Trotov M, Kuznetsov D. ICM - A new method for protein modeling and design: applications to docking and structure prediction from the distorted native conformation. J. Comput.Chem., 1994, 15: 488-506.

[311] Totrov M, Abagyan, R. Flexible protein-ligand docking by global energy optimization in internal coordinates. Proteins: Struct., Funct., Bioinform., 1997, 29: 215-220.

[312] Koshland DEJ. The key-lock theory and the induced fit theory. Angew. Chem. Int. Ed. Engl., 1994, 33: 2408-2412.

[313] Creighton TE. Proteins: Structures and Molecular Properties, W. H. Freeman and Company: New York, 1993. Fischer, E. Einfluss der Configuration auf die Wirkung der Enzyme.BerDtsch Chem. Ges. 1894, 27: 2985-2993.

[314] Lichtenthaler FW. 100 Years "Schluessel-Schloss-Prinzip": what made Emil Fischer use this analogy? Angew. Chem. Int. Ed. Engl. 1995, 33: 2364-2374.

[315] Bosshard HR. Molecular recognition by induced fit: how fit is the concept? News Physiol. Sci., 2001, 16: 171-173.

[316] Freire E. Statistical thermodynamic linkage between conformational and binding equilibria. Adv. Protein Chem., 1998, 51: 255- 279.

[317] Ma B, Kumar S, Tsai CJ, Nussinov R. Folding funnels and binding mechanisms. Protein Eng., 1999, 12: 713-720.

[318] Gunasekaran K, Ma B, Nussinov R. Is allostery an intrinsic property of all dynamic proteins? Proteins: Struct., Funct., Bioinform., 2004, 57: 433-443.

[319] Xu Y, Colletier JP, Jiang H, Silman I, Sussman JL, Weik M. Induced-fit or preexisting equilibrium dynamics? Lessons from protein crystallography and MD simulations on acetylcholinesterase and implications for structure-based drug design. Protein Sci., 2008, 17: 601-605.

[320] Hammes GG, Chang YC, Oas TG. Conformational selection or induced fit: a flux description of reaction mechanism. Proc. Natl. Acad. Sci. USA, 2009, 106: 13737-13741.

]321] Peng S, Lin X, Cho Z, Huang N, Identifying multiple-target ligands *via* computational chemogenomics approaches, Current Topics in medicinal chemistry, 2012,12:1363-1375.

[322] Ma XH, Shi Z, Tan C, Jiang Y, Go ML, Low BC, Chen YZ, In-silico approaches to multi-target drug discovery:computer aided multi-target drug design, multi-target virtual screening, Pharm. Res, 2010, 27: 739-749.

[323] Dik-Lung Ma DL Chana DSH and Leung CH, Drug repositioning by structure-based virtual screening, Chem. Soc. Rev., 2013, 42: 2130—2141.

[324] Ghemtio L, Pérez-Nueno VI, Leroux V, Asses Y, Souchet M, Mavridis L, Maigret B and W. Ritchie DW, RDeng, Z.; Chuaqui, C.; Singh, J. Recent trends and applications in 3d virtual screening, Combinatorial Chemistry and high-throughput screening, 2012:15:749-769.

[325] Deng Z, Chuaqui C, Singh J. Knowledge-based design of target focused libraries using protein-ligand interaction constraints. J. Med. Chem., 2006, 49: 490-500.

[326] Li L, Wang B, Meroueh SO. Support vector regression scoring of receptor-ligand complexes for rank-ordering and virtual screening of chemical libraries. J. Chem. Inf. Model., 2011, 51: 2132-2138.

[327] Xue MZ, Zheng MY, Xiong B, Li YL, Jiang HL Shen JK. Knowledge-Based Scoring Functions in Drug Design. Developing a Target-Specific Method for Kinase-Ligand Interactions. J. Chem. Inf. Model., 2010, 50: 1378-1386.

[328] Ghemtio L, Devignes MD, Smaïl-Tabbone M, Souchet M, Leroux V, Maigret B. Comparison of three preprocessing filters efficiency in virtual screening: identification of new putative LXRß regulators as a test case. J. Chem. Inf. Model., 2010, 50: 701-715.

[329] Seoud RA. Bio HCVKD: a bioinformatics knowledge discovery system for HCV drug discovery-identifying proteins, ligands and active residues, in biological literature. Int. J. Bioinform. Res. App., 2011, 7: 317-333.

[330] Medina-Aunon JA, Paradela A, Macht M, Thiele H, Corthals G, Albar JP. Protein information and knowledge extractor: Discovering biological information from proteomics data. Proteomics, 2010, 10: 3262-3271.

[331] Zheng MY, Xiong B, Luo C, Li S, Liu X, Shen QC, Li J, Zhu W L, Luo XM, Jiang H L. Knowledge-based scoring functions in drug design: 3. A two-dimensional knowledge based hydrogen-bonding potential for the prediction of protein ligand interactions. J. Chem. Inf. Model., 2011, 51: 2994-3004.

[332] Shen QC, Xiong B, Zheng MY, Luo XM, Luo C, Liu XA, Du Y, Li J, Zhu WL, Shen J. K, Jiang HL. Knowledgebased scoring functions in drug design: 2. Can the knowledge base be enriched? J. Chem. Inf. Model., 2011, 51: 386-397.

[333] Ghose AK, Herbertz T, Salvino JM.; Mallamo JP. Knowledge-based chemoinformatic approaches to drug discovery.Drug Discov. Today, 2006, 11: 1107-1114.

[334] Hristovski D, Daeroski S, Peterlin B, Roi-Hristovski A. Supporting discovery in medicine by association rule mining of bibliographic databases. Stud. Health Technol. Inform., 2001, 84: 1344-1348.

[335] Ghose AK, Herbertz T, Hudkins RL, Dorsey BD, Mallamo JP. Knowledge-based, central nervous system (CNS) lead selection and lead optimization for CNS drug discovery. ACS Chem. neurosci., 2012, 3: 50-68.

[336] Ghose AK, Herbertz T, Pippin DA, Salvino JM, Mallamo JP. Knowledge based prediction of ligand binding modes and rational inhibitor design for kinase drug discovery. J. Med. Chem., 2008, 51: 5149-5171.

[337] Simmons K, Kinney J, Owens A, Kleier DA, Bloch K, Argentar D, Walsh A, Vaidyanathan G. Practical outcomes of applying ensemble machine learning classifiers to High-Throughput Screening (HTS) data analysis and screening. J. Chem. Inf. Model., 2008, 48: 2196-2206.

[338] Blundell TL, Sibanda BL, Sternberg MJ, Thornton JM. Knowledge-based prediction of protein structures and the design of novel molecules. Nature, 1987, 326:347-352

[339] Parenti MD, Rastelli G, Advances and applications of binding affinity prediction methods in drug discovery, Biotechnology Advances, 2012, 30: 244-250.

[340] de Azevedo WF, Dias R. Computational methods for calculation of ligand-binding affinity. Curr. Drug Targets. 2008, 9: 1031-1039.

[341] Jorgensen WJ. Efficient drug lead discovery and optimization. Acc. Chem. Res. 2009, 42: 724-733.

[342] Yuriev E and Ramsland PA, Latest developments in molecular docking : 2010-2011 in review. J. Mol. Recognition, 2013, 26:215-239.

[343] Wang W, He W, Zhou X and Chen X. Optimization of molecular docking scores with support vector rank regression. Proteins. 2013, 81:1386-1398.

[344] Zheng Z and Merz Jr. KM. Development of the knowledge-based and empirical combined scoring algorithm (KECSA) to score protein-ligand interactions. Chem. Inf. And modeling. 2013, 53:1073-1083.

[345] Fan H, Schneidman-Duhovny DS, Irwin JJ, Dong G, Shoichet BK and Sali A, Statistical potential for modeling and ranking of protein-ligand interactions. Chemical Information and Modeling, 2011,51:3078-3092.

[346] Durant JD, Friedman AJ, Rogers KE and McCammon JA. Comparing neural-network scoring functions and the state of the art: Applications to common library screening. Chemical Informatin and modeling, J. Chem. Informaiton and modeling,2013,53:726-1735.

[347] Liu J, He X and Zhang JZH. Improving the scoring of protein-ligand binding affinity by including the effects of structural water and electronic polarization. Chemical information and modeling, 2013,53:1306-1314.

[348] Sastry GM, Inakolly VSS and Sherman W, Boosting virtual screening enrichments with data fusion:Coalescing hits from two-dimensional fingerprints, shape and docking. J. Chem. Information and Modeling. 2013, 53:1531-1542.

[349] Korb O, McCabe P, Cole J. The ensemble performance index: An improved measure for assessing ensemble pose prediction performance. J. Chem. Information and Modeling, 2011, 51:2915-2919.

[350] Guimaraes CRW. A direct comparison of the MM-GB/SA scoring procedure and free-energy perturbation calculations using carbonic anhydrase as a test case: strengths and pitfalls of each compound, J. of Chemical Theory and Computation, 2011,7:2296-2306.

[351] Liu Yl and Wang R. Test MM-PB/SA on true conformational ensembles of protein-ligand complexes, J. Chem. In. Model. 2010, 50: 1682-1692.

[352] Xiang M, Cao Y, Fan W, Chen L and Mo Y Compuer-aided drug design:Lead discovery and optimizations, Combinatorial chemistry & high throughput screening, 2012, 15:328-337.

[353] Gohike H, Klebe G. Approaches to the description and prediction of the leading binding affinity of small-molecule ligands to macromolecular receptors. Angew. Chem. Int. Ed. 2002, 41, 15:2644-2676.

[354] Song CH, Lim SJ and Tang JC, Recent advances in computer-aided drug design, Briefings in bioinformatics, 2009, 10:579-591.

[355] Huang SY, Grinter SZ and Zou X, Scoring functions and their evaluation methods for protein-ligand docking: recent advances and future directions, Phys. Chem Chem. Phys 2010,12:12899-12098.

[356] Kawatkar S, Mustakas D, Miller M and McCarthy DJ, Virtual fragment screening: exploration of MM-PBSA rescoring, J. Comput. Aided Mol. Des. 2013, 26:921-914.

[357] Wang W, He W, Zhou X and Chen X, Optimization of molecular docking score with support vector rank regression, Proteins, 2013, 81: 1386-1398.

[358] Hsieh JH, Yin S, Wang XS, Liu, Dokholyan NV and Tropsha A, Chemoinformatics meets molecular mechanics: A combined application of knowledge-based pose scoring and physical force field-based hit scoring functions improves the accuracy of structure-based virtual screening. J. Chem. Inf. And Model. 2012, 52: 16-28.

[359] Fan H, Schneidman-Duhovny D, Irwin JJ, Dong G, Shoichet BK and Sali A, Statistical potential for modeling and ranking of protein-ligand interactions, J. Chem. Information and Modeling, 2011, 51:3078-3092.

[360] Pauli dos Santos RN, Rostirolla DC, Martinelli LK, Ducati RG, Timmers LFSM, Basso LA, Santos DS, Guido RVC, Andricopulo AD and de Souza ON, Discovery of new inhibitors of mycobacterium tuberculosis enzyme using virtual screening and a 3d-pharmacophore-based approach, J. Chem. Inf. and modeling, 2013,43: 2390-2401.

[361] Ma XH, Zhu F, Liu X, Shi Z, Zhang JX, Yang SY, Wei YQ and Chen YZ. Virtual screening methods as tools for drug lead discovery from large chemical libraries, Current medicinal chemistry, 2012, 19: 5562-5571.

[362] Christ CD, Mark AE, van Gunsteren WF. Basic ingredients of the free energy calculations: a review. J. Comput. Chem. 2010, 31: 1469-1582.

[363] Deng Y, Roux B. Computations of standard binding free energies with molecular dynamics simulations. J. Phys Chem. B, 2009, 113: 2245-2246.

[364] Phillips JC, Braun R, Wang W, Gumbart J, Tajkorshid E, Villa E, Chipot C, Skeel RD, Kale L, Schulten K. Scalable molecular dynamics with NAMD. J. Comput. Chem. 2005, 26:1781-1802.

[365] DiMaio F, Terwilliger TC, Read RJ, Wlodaver A, Oberdorfer G, Wagner U,Valikov E, Alon A, Fass D, Axelrod HL, Das D, Vorobiev SM, Iwai H, Pokkuluri PR, Baker D. Improved molecular replacement by density-and energy-guided protein structure optimization. Nature, 2011, 473: 540-543.

[366] Taft CA, Silva CHTP, State of the art in quantum mechanics based methods in drug design, Chapter 1, New developments in Medicinal Chemistry, Bentham Science Publishers, 2010 Eds. (Bentham Science, U.A.E.) pp 1-56.

[367] Ball P. Water as an active constituent in cell biology. Chem. Rev 2008, 108:74-108.

[368]   Homans SW. Water, water everywhere-except where it matters?, Drug Discov. Today, 2007, 12:534-539.

[369]   Paesani F, 371Voth GA. The properties of water: insights from quantum simulations. J. Phys. Chem. B, 2009,113: 5702-5719.

[370]   Chong, SH, Ham S. Interaction with the Surrounding Water Plays a Key Role in Determining the Aggregation Propensity of Proteins. Angewandte Chemie, International, 2014, 53:3961-3964.

[371]   Valérie Vallet1, Jean-Pierre Flament1 and Michel Masella2, Revisiting a many-body model for water based on a single polarizable site: From gas phase clusters to liquid and air/liquid water systems, J. Chem. Phys. 2013, 139: 114502.

[372]   Kirchmair J, Spitzer GM, Liedl KR. Considerationof water and solvation effects in virtual screening. In virtual screening principles, challenges and practical guidelines, Scriffer CA, Ed. Wiley-VCH Verlag: 2011, pp 263-289.

[373]   Barillari C, Taylor J, Viner R Essex JW, Classification of water molecules in protein binding sites. J. Am. Chem. Soc. 2007, 129: 2577-2587.

[374]   Zahou T, Huang D, Caflish A. Quantum mechanical methods for drug design. Curr. Top. Med. Chem. 2010, 10:33-45.

[375]   Spiegela K, Magistrato A. Modeling anticancer drug-DNA interactions *via* mexed QM/MM molecular dynamics simulations. Org. Biomol. Chem. 2006, 4: 2507-2517.

[376]   Senn HM, Thiel W. QM/MM methods for biomolecular systems Angew. Chem. Int. Ed. 2009, 48:1198-1229.

[377]   Menikarachchi LC, Gascon JA, QM/MM approaches in medicinal chemistry research. Curr. Top. Med. Chem. 2010, 10: 46-54.

[378]   Glao J, Amara P, Alhambra C, Field MJ. A generalized hybrid orbital (GHO) method for the treatment of boundary atoms in combined QM/MM calculations. J. Phys. Chem. A. 1998, 102:4714-4721.

[379]   Friesner RA. Combined quantum and molecular mechanics (QM/MM). Drug Disc. Today, 2004, 1: 253-260.

[380]   Alzate-Morales JH, Contreras R, Soriano A, Tunon I, Silla E. A computational study of the protein-ligand interaction in CDK2 inhibitors: using quantum mechanics/molecular mechanics interaction energy as a predictor of the biological activity. Biophys. J. 2007, 92: 430-439.

[381]   Willett P. Similarity-based virtual screening using 2D fingerprints. Drug Discovery Today, 2006, 11: 1046-1053.

[382]   Satry M, Lowne JF, Dixon SL, Sherman W. Large-scale systematic analysis of 2D fingerprint methods and parameters to improve virtual screening enrichments. J. Chem. Inf. Model. 2010, 50: 771-784.

[383]   Duan JX, Dixon SL, Lowrie JF, Sherman W. Analysis and comparison of 2D fingerprints: Insights into database screening performance using eight fingerprint methods. J. Mol. Graphics. Model. 2010, 20: 157-170.

[384]   Schuffenhauer A, Gillet VJ, Willen P. Similarity searching in files of three-dimensional chemical structure analysis of the BIOSTER database using two-dimensional fingerprints and molecular field descriptors. J. Chem. Inf. Comput. Sci. 2000, 40: 295-307.

[385]   Cheeseright TJ, Mackey MD, Melville JL, Vinter JG. FieldScreen: virtual screening using molecular fields: Application to the DUD data set J. Chem. Inf. Model. 2008, 48: 2108-2117.

[386]   Kearsley SK, Smith GM. An alternative method for the alignment of molecular structures: Maximizing electrostatic and steric overlap. Tetrahedron Comput.Meth. 1990, 3: 615-653.

[387] Brooijmans N and Kuntz ID. Molecular recognition and docking algorithms. Annual Review of Biophysics and Biomolecular Structure.2003, 32: 335-373.

[388] Ebalunoide JO, Ouyang Z, Liang J, Zheng W. Novel approach to structure-based pharmacophore search using computational geometry and shape matching techniques. J. Chem. Inf. Model. 2008, 48: 889-901.

[389] Brown N, Jacoby E. On scaffolds and hopping in medicinal chemistry. Mini Rev. Med. Chem. 2006, 6: 1217-1219.

[390] Proschak E, Rupp M, Derksen S, Schneider G, Shapelets: Possibilities and limitation of shape-based virtual screening. J. Comput. Chem. 2008, 29: 108-114.

[391] Vainio MJ, Puranen JS, Johnson MS. ShaEP: molecular overlay based on shape and electrostatic potential. J. Chem. Inf. Model. 2009, 49: 492-502.

[392] Grant JA, Gallardo MA, Pickup BT, A fast method of molecular shape comparison: a simple application of the Gaussian description of molecular shape. J. Comput. Chem. 1996, 17: 1653-1660.

[393] Rush TS, Grant JA, Morsysk L, Nicholls A. A shape-based 3-D scaffold hoppin method and its application to a bacterial protein-protein interaction. J. Med. Chem. 2005, 48, 1489-1495.

[394] Mavridis L, Hudson BD, Richie DW. Toward high throuput 3D virtual screening using spherical harmonic surface representations. J. Chem. Inf. Model. 2007, 47: 1787-1796.

[395] Cai W, Shao X, Maigret B. Protein-ligand recognition using spherical harmonic molecular surfaces: towards a fast and efficient filter for large virtual throughput screening. J. Mol. Graph. Model. 2002, 20: 313-328.

[396] Ritchie DW, Kemp GJL. Protein docking using spherical polar Fourier correlations Proteins. 2000, 39: 178-194.

[397] Henrich S, Salo-Ahen OMH, Huang B, Rippmann FF, Cruciani G, Wade RC. Computational approaches to identifying and characterizing protein binding site for ligand design J. Mol. Recognit. 2010, 23: 209-219.

[398] Gold ND, Jackson RM, SitesBase: a database for structure-based protein-ligand binding site comparisons. Nucleic Acids Res. 2006, 34: D231-D234.

[399] Yang L, Chen J, Shi L, Hudock MP, Wang K, He L. Identifying unexpected therapeutic target *via* chemical-protein interactions. PLoSOne, 2010,5: 9568-9571.

[400] Kirkpatrick P, Ellis C, Chemical space. Nature, 2004, 432:823-823

[401] Lipkus AH, Yuan Q, Lucas KA, Funk SA, Bartlett III WF, Schenck RJ, Trippe AJ. Structural diversity of organic chemistry. A scaffold analysis of the CAS registry, J. Org. Chem 2008, 73: 443-445.

[402] Sanderson CM, The cartographers toolbox: building bigger and better human protein interaction networks. Brief Funct Genomic Proteomic, 2009, 8: 1-11.

[403] Ritchie DW, Recent progress and future directions in protein-protein docking. Curr Protein Pept Sci, 2008, 9: 1-15.

[404] Kastritis PL, Bonvin AM (2010) Are scoring functions in protein-protein docking ready to predict interactomes? Clues from a novel binding affinity benchmark. J Proteome Res, 2010, 9: 2216-25.

[405] Andrusier N, Mashiach E, Nussinov R, Wolfson HJ, Principles of flexible protein-protein docking. Proteins, 2008, 73: 271-89.

[406] Bernauer J, Bahadur RP, Rodier F, Janin J, Poupon A. DiMoVo: A Voronoi tessellation based method for discriminating crystallographic and biological protein-protein interactions. Bioinformatics, 2008, 24: 652-658.

[407] Bernauer J, Poupon A, Aze J, Janin J. A docking analysis of the statistical physics of protein-protein recognition. Phys Biol, 2005, 2: S17-S23.

[408] Bernauer J, Aze J, Janin J, Poupon A. A new protein-protein docking scoring function based on interface residue properties. Bioinformatics, 2007, 23: 555-562.

[409] Lensink MF, Mendez R, Wodak SJ, Docking and scoring protein complexes: CAPRI 3rd Edition. Proteins, 2007, 69: 704-718.

[410] Mendez R, Leplae R, Lensink MF, Wodak SJ. Assessment of CAPRI predictions in rounds 3-5 shows progress in docking procedures. Proteins, 2005, 60:150-69.

[411] De Las Rivas J and Fontanillo C, Protein-protein interaction networks: unraveling the wiring of molecular machines within the cell, Briefings in functional genomics, 2012, 2:489-496.

[412] Vajda S, Hall DR and Kozakov D, Sampling and scoring: a marriage made in heaven, 2013, 81, 1874-1884.

[413] Hook LA, Stem cell technology for drug discovery and development, Drug Discovery Today, 2012, 17: 336-342.

[414] Alison MR and Islam S. Attributes of adult stem cells. J. Pathol. 2009, 217:144-1460.

[415] Copelan EA, Hematopoietic stem-cell transplantation. N. Engl. J. Med., 2006, 354:1813-1826.

[416] Czechowicz, A. and Weissman, IL. Purified hematopoietic stem cell transplantation: the next generation of blood and immune replacement. Immunol. Allergy Clin. North Am. 2010, 30: 159-171

[417] Ruin LL and Haston KM. Stem cell biology and drug discovery. BMC Biol., 2011, 9: 42-43.

[418] Clark DE, What has virtual screening ever done for drug discovery? Exp. Opin. Drug Discov., 2008, 3: 841-851.

[419] Shoichet, B. K. Virtual screening of chemical libraries. Nature, 2004, 432; 862-865.

[420] Bajorath J. Integration of virtual and high-throughput screening. Nat. Rev. Drug Discov. 2002, 1: 882-894.

[421] Mestres J. Virtual screening: a real screening complement to highthroughput screening. Biochem. Soc. Trans., 2002, 30: 797-799.

[422] Phatak SS, Stephan CC, Cavasotto CN. High-throughput and *in silico* screenings in drug discovery. Exp. Opin. Drug Discov., 2009, 4: 947-959.

[423] Davies JW, Glick M, Jenkins JL. Streamlining lead discovery by aligning *in silico* and high-throughput screening. Curr. Opin. Chem. Biol., 2006, 10: 343-351.

[424] Hawkins PCD, Skillman AG, Nicholls A. Comparison of shape-matching and docking as virtual screening tools. J. Med. Chem., 2007, 50: 74-82.

[425] Tanrikulu Y, Schneider G. Pseudoreceptor models in drug design: bridging ligand- and receptor-based virtual screening. Nat. Rev. Drug Discov., 2008, 7: 667-677.

[426] Clark RD. Prospective ligand- and target-based 3D QSAR: state of the art 2008. Curr. Top. Med. Chem., 2009, 9: 791-810.

[427] Koutsoukas A, Simms B,Kirchmair J, Bond PJ, Whitmore AV, Zimmer S, Young MP, Jenkins JL, Glick M, Glen RC. Bender, A. From *in silico* target prediction to multi-target drug design: Current databases, methods and applications. J. Proteomics, 2011, 74: 2554-2574.

[428] Omagari K, Mitomo D, Kubota S, Nakamura H, Fukunishi Y. A method to enhance the hit ratio by a combination of structurebased drug screening and ligand-based screening. Adv. Appl. Bioinform. Chem., 2008, 1: 19-28.

[429] Villoutreix BO, Renault N, Lagorce D, Sperandio O,Montes M, Miteva MA. Free resources to assist structure-based virtual ligand screening experiments. Curr. Protein Pept. Sci., 2007, 8: 381-411.

[430] Leeson PD, St-Gallay SA. The influence of the 'organizational factor' on compound quality in drug discovery. Nat. Rev. Drug Discov. 2011, 10: 749-765.

[431] Michel J, Essex JW. Prediction of protein-ligand binding affinity by free energy simulations: assumptions, pitfalls and expectations. J. Comp. Aided Mol Des. 2010, 24: 639-658.

[432] Munos B. Lessons from 60 years of pharmaceutical innovation. Nat. Rev. Drug Discov., 2009, 8: 959-968.

[433] Schmid EF, Smith DA. Is declining innovation in the pharmaceutical industry a myth? Drug Discov. Today, 2005, 10: 1031-1039.

[434] Williams R. Discontinued drugs in 2008: oncology drugs. Exp. Opin. Invest. Drugs, 2009, 18: 1581-1594.

[435] Harrison C. The patent cliff steepens. Nat. Rev. Drug Discov. 2011, 10: 12-13.

[436] LaMattina JL. The impact of mergers on pharmaceutical R&D. Nat. Rev. Drug Discov., 2011, 10: 559-560.

[437] Tralau-Stewart CJ, Wyatt CA, Kleyn DE, Ayad A. Drug discovery: new models for industry-academic partnerships. Drug Discov. Today, 2009, 14: 95-101.

[438] Triggle DJ. The chemist as astronaut: searching for biologically useful space in the chemical universe. Biochem. Pharmacol., 2009, 78: 217-223.

[439] Irwin JJ. Staring off into chemical space. Nat. Chem. Biol., 2009, 5: 536-537.

[440] Knox C, Law V, Jewison T, Liu P, Ly S, Frolkis A, Pon A, Banco K, Mak C, Neveu V, Djoumbou Y, Eisner R, Guo AC, Wishart DS. DrugBank 3.0: a comprehensive resource for 'omics' research on drugs. Nucleic Acids Res., 2011, 39: D1035-D1041.

[441] Koutsoukas A, Simms B, Kirchmair J, Bond PJ, Whitmore AV, Zimmer S, Young M P, Jenkins JL, Glick M, Glen RC, Bender A. From in *silico* target prediction to multi-target drug design: current databases, methods and applications. J. Proteomics, 2011, 74: 2554-2574.

[442] Koppen H. Virtual screening - what does it give us? Curr. Opin. Drug Discov. Develop., 2009, 12: 397-407.

[443] Caldwell GW. Compound optimization in early- and late-phase drug discovery: acceptable pharmacokinetic properties utilizing combined physicochemical, *in vitro* and *in vivo* screens. Curr. Opin. Drug Discov. Develop., 2000, 3: 30-41.

[444] Raju TNK. The Nobel chronicles. The Lancet, 2000, 356: 346.

[445] DiMasi JA, Faden LB. Competitiveness in follow-on drug R&D: a race or imitation? Nat. Rev. Drug Discov., 2011, 10: 23-27.

[446] Sundar S, Jha TK, Thakur CP, Bhattacharya SK, Rai M. Oral miltefosine for the treatment of Indian visceral leishmaniasis. T. Roy. Soc. Trop. Med. H, 2006, 100S: 26-33.

[447] Wermuth CG. Selective optimization of side activities: another way for drug discovery. J. Med. Chem., 2004, 47: 1303-1314.

[448] Congreve M, Chessari G, Tisi D. Woodhead, A. J. Recent developments in fragment-based drug discovery. J. Med. Chem., 2008, 51: 3661-3680.

[449] Pérez-Nueno VI, Ritchie DW, Borrell JI, Teixidó J. Clustering and classifying diverse HIV entry inhibitors using a novel consensus shape-based virtual screening approach: further evidence for multiple binding sites within the CCR5 extracellular pocket. J. Chem. Inf. Model., 2008, 48: 2146-2165.

[450] Pérez-Nueno VI, Ritchie DW, Rabal O, Pascual R, Borrell JI, Teixidó J. Comparison of ligand-based and receptor-based virtual screening of HIV entry inhibitors for the CXCR4 and CCR5 receptors using 3D ligand shape matching and ligand-receptor docking. J. Chem. Inf. Model., 2008, 48: 509-533.

[451] Cai W, Xu J, Shao X, Leroux V, Beautrait A, Maigret B. SHEF: a vHTS geometrical filter using coefficients of spherical harmonic molecular surfaces. J. Mol. Model., 2008, 14: 393-401.

[452] Beautrait A, Leroux V, Chavent M, Ghemtio L, Devignes MD, Smaïl-Tabbone M, Cai W, Shao X, Moreau G, Bladon P, Yao J, Maigret B. Multiple-step virtual screening using VSMG:overview and validation of fast geometrical matching enrichment. J. Mol. Model., 2008, 14: 135-148.

[453] Moitessier N, Englebienne P, Lee D, Lawandi J, Corbeil CR. Towards the development of universal, fast and highly accurate docking/scoring methods: a long way to go. Br. J. Pharmacol. 2008, 153: S7-S26.

[454] Warren GL, Andrews CW, Capelli AM, Clarke B, LaLonde J, Lambert MH, Lindvall M, Nevins N, Semus SF, Senger S, Tedesco G, Wall ID, Woolven JM, Peishoff CE, Head M S. A critical assessment of docking programs and scoring functions. J. Med. Chem., 2006, 49: 5912-5931.

[455] Kellenberger E, Rodrigo J, Muller P, Rognan D. Comparative evaluation of eight docking tools for docking and virtual screening accuracy. Proteins, 2004, 57: 225-242.

[456] Cozzini, P, Kellogg GE, Spyrakis F, Abraham DJ, Costantino G, Emerson A, Fanelli F.; Gohlke H, Kuhn LA, Morris GM, Orozco M, Pertinhez TA, Rizzi M, Sotriffer CA. Target flexibility: an emerging consideration in drug discovery and design. J. Med. Chem., 2008, 51: 6237-6255.

[457] Beautrait A, Leroux V, Chavent M, Ghemtio L, Devignes MD, Smaïl-Tabbone M, Cai, W, Shao X, Moreau G, Bladon P, Yao J, Maigret B. Multiple-step virtual screening using VSMG: overview and validation of fast geometrical matching enrichment. J. Mol. Model., 2008, 14: 135-148.

[458] Cannon EO, Nigsch F,Mitchell JBO. A novel hybrid ultrafast shape descriptor method for use in virtual screening. Chem. Cent. J., 2008, 2: 3-5.

[459] Tiwari A, Sekhar AK. Workflow based framework for life science informatics. Comput. Biol. Chem., 2007, 31: 305-319.

[460] Berthold MR, Cebron N, Dill F, Gabriel TR, Kötter T, Meinl T, Ohl P, Thiel K, Wiswedel B. KNIME - The Konstanz Information Miner. SIGKDD Explorations, 2008, 11: 26-31.

[461] Pipeline Pilot Accelrys Inc., San Diego, CA, USA.

[462 Hassan M, Brown RD, Varma-O'brien S, Rogers D. Cheminformatics analysis and learning in a data pipelining environment. Mol. Divers, 2006, 10: 283-99.

[463] Ghemtio L, Smail-Tabbone M, Devignes MD, Souchet M, Maigret B. In: *A KDD approach for designing filtering strategies to improve virtual screening*, Procedings of the KDIR International Conference on Knowledge Discovery and Information Retrieval, Madeira, Portugal, 2009-10-06, 2009-10-09; F. Ana, Ed; INSTIC: Madeira, Portugal, **2009**.

[464] Rodrigues MO, de Paula MV, Wanderley KA, Iane B. Vasconcelos IB, Severino Alves, Jr., and Soares TA, Metal Organic Frameworks for Drug Delivery and Environmental Remediation: A Molecular Docking Approach Journal of Quantum Chemistry 2012, 112: 3346-3355.

[465] Ebejer JP, Fulle S, Morris GM and Finn PW, The emerging role of cloud computing in molecular modeling. J. of molecular graphics and modeling. 2013, 44: 177-187.

[466] P. Mell, T. Grance, The NIST definition of cloud computing, NIST Special Publication 2011, 800: 145.

[467] Vaquero LM, Rodero-Merino, J. Caceres, Lindner M, A break in the clouds:towards a cloud definition, ACM SIGCOMM Computer Communication Review. 2009, 39: 50-55.

[468] Marston S, Li Z, Bandyopadhyay S, Zhang J, Ghalsasi A, Cloud computing—the business perspective, Decision Support Systems. 2011, 51: 176-189.

[469] Buyya R, Yeo CS, Venugopal S, Broberg J, Brandic I, Cloud computing and emerging IT platforms: vision, hype, and reality for delivering computing as the 5th utility, Future Generation Computer Systems. 2009, 25: 599-616.

[470] R.L. Grossman, The case for cloud computing, IT Professional. 2009, 11: 23-27.

[471] Mateescu G, Gentzsch W, Ribbens CJ, Hybrid computing—where HPC meets grid and cloud computing, Future Generation Computer Systems. 2011, 27: 440-453.

[472] Marinos A, G. Briscoe, Community cloud computing, Cloud Computing. 2009, 47:2-484.

[473] Dean J, Ghemawat S, MapReduce: simplified data processing on large clusters, Communications of the ACM. 2008, 51: 107-113.

[474] Foster I, Zhao Y, Raicu I, Lu S, Cloud computing and grid computing 360- degree compared, in: Grid Computing Environments Workshop, 2008. GCE'08, 2008, pp. 1-10.

[475] Gong C, Liu J, Zhang Q, Chen H, Gong Z, The characteristics of cloud computing, in: Parallel Processing Workshops (ICPPW), 2010 39th International Conference on, IEEE, 2010, pp. 257-259.

[476] Armbrust M, Fox A, Griffith R, Joseph AD, Katz R, Konwinski A, *et al.*, A view of cloud computing, Communications of the ACM. 2010, 53: 50-58.

[477] Nurmi D, Wolski R, Grzegorczyk C, Obertelli G, Soman S, Youseff L *et al.*, The eucalyptus open-source cloud-computing system, in: 9th IEEE/ACM International Symposium on Cluster Computing and the Grid, 2009, pp. 124-131.

[478] Armstrong MS, Morris GM, Finn PW, Sharma R, Moretti L, Cooper RI, *et al.*, ElectroShape: fast molecular similarity calculations incorporating shape, chirality and electrostatics, Journal of Computer-Aided Molecular Design. 2010, 24: 789-801.

[479] Barbosa AJM and Del Rio A, Freely accessible databases of commercial compounds for high-throughput virtual screenings, Current topics in medicinal chemistry, 2012, 12:866-877.

[480] Li R, Bajorath J, Systematic assessment of scaffold distances in ChEMBL: prioritizaition of compound data sets for scaffold hopping analysis in virtual screening, J. Comput. Aided Mol Des., 2012, 26: 1101-1109.

[481] Del Rio A, Barbosa A, Caporuscio F. Use of large multiconformational databases with structure-based pharmacophore models for fast screening of commercial compound collections. J. Chem Inform. 2011, 3: 27-31.

[482] Schneider G. Virtual screening: an endless staircase? Nat. Rev. Drug. Discov. 2010, 9: 273-276.

[483] Weininger D. SMILES, a chemical language and information system. Introduction to methodology and encoding rules. J. Chem. Inf. Comput. Sci 1988, 28: 31-36.

[484]   Thalleim T, Vollmer A, Ebert Ru, Kuhne R, Schuurmann G. Tautomer identification and tautomer structure generation based on the InChI Code. J. Chem. Inf. Model. 2010, 50:1223-1232.

[485]   ten Brink T, Exner TE. Influence of protonation, tautomeric and stereoisomeric states on protein-ligand docking results. J. Chem. Inf. Model. 2009, 49: 1535-1546.

[486]   Lipinski CA, Lombardo F, Dominy BW, Feeney PJ. Experimental and computational approaches to estimate solubility and permeability in drug discovery and development settings. Adv. Drug Delivery Rev. 2001, 46:3-26.

[487]   Stouch TR, The errors of our ways: taking account of error in computer-aided drug design to build confidence intervals for our next 25 years, J. Comput. Aided Mol. Des. 2012, 26:125-134.

[488]   Carlson HA, Dunbar JB. A call to arms: what you can do for computational drug discovery. J. Chem. Inf. Model, 2011, 51:2025-2026.

[489]   Guthrie JP. A blind challenge for computational solvation free energies: introduction and overview. J. Phys. Chem. B, 2009, 113:4501-4507.

[490]   Muchmore SW, Debe DA, Metz JT, Brown SP, Martin YC, Hajduk PJ, 2008. Application ofbelief theory to similarity data fusion for use in analog searching and lead hopping. J. Chem. Inf. Mode. 2008, 48: 941-948.

[491]   Tejwani RW, Davis ME, Anderson BD, Stouch TR, An atomic and molecular view of the depth dependence of the free energies of solute transfer from water into lipid bilayers. 2011, Mol. Phar, 2011, 8: 2204-2215.

[492]   Friesner RA, Banks JL, Murphy RB, Halgren TA, Klicic JJ, Mainz DT, Repasky MP, Knoll EH, Shaw DE,Shelley M, Perry JK, Francis P, Shenkin PS, "Glide: A New Approach for Rapid, Accurate Docking and Scoring. 1. Method and Assessment of Docking Accuracy", J. Med. Chem. 2004, 47, 1739-1749.

[493]   Jones G, Willett P, Glen RC, Molecular recognition of receptor sites using a genetic algorithm with a description of desolvation. J. Mol. Biol, 1995, 245:43-53.

[494]   Venkatachalam CM, Jian X, Oldfield T, Waldman MJ, LigandFit: a novel method for the shape-directed rapid docking of ligands to protein active sites. Mol. Graph Model 2003, 21: 289-307.

[495]   Ravitz O, Zsoldos Z, Simon A, Improving molecular docking through eHITS turntable scoring functiron, J. Comput. Aided Mol. Design, 2011, 25:1033-1051.

[496]   Rarey M, Kramer B, Lengauer T and Klebe GA, A fast flexible docking method using incremental construction algorithm, J. Mol. Biology, 1996, 261:470-489.

[497]   Gann M, FRED Pose prediction and virtual screening accuracy, Chemical Information and Modeling, 2011, 51:578-596.

[498]   McGann M, FRED and HYBRID docking performance on standardized dataset, J. Comput Aided Mol. Des., 2012, 26: 897-906.

[499]   Splitzer R, Jain AN, Surflex-Dock: Docking benchmarks and real-world application, J. Comput. Aided Mol. Des. 2012, 26: 687-699.

[500]   Dakshanamurthy S, Issa NT, Assefnia S, Seshasayee A, Peters OJ, Madhavan S, Uren A, Brown ML and Byers SW. Predicting new indications for approved drugs using a proteochemometric method, Journal of Medicinal Chemistry, 2012, 55:6832-6848.

[501]   Klenner A, Weisel M, Reisen F, Proschak E and Schneider G, Automated docking of flexible molecules into receptor binding sites by ligand self-organizaion *in situ*, Mol Info, 2010, 29:189-193.

[502]   Hubbard RE, Davis B, Chen I and Drysdale MJ, The SeeDs approach: Integrating fragments into drug discovery, Current topics in medicinal chemistry, 2007, 7:1568-1581.

[503] Trott O, Olson AJ, Docking with a new scoring function, Efficient optimization and multithreading, J. Comput. Chem, 2010, 31:455-461

[504] Grosdidier A, Zoete V, Michielin O, Fast docking using the CHARMM force field with EADock DSS, J. Comput. Chem, 2011, 32:2149-2159.

[505] Zavodsky MI, Sanschagrin PC, Korde RS, Kuhn LA, Distilling the essential features of a protein surface for improving protein-ligand docking, scoring and virtual screening, J. Comput. Aided Mol. Des. 2002, 16: 883 - 902.

[506] Qian L,Brian M, Karl S and Julian S. Tagged Fragment Method for Evolutionary Structure-Based *De Novo* Lead Generation and Optimization, J. Med. Chem. 2007, 50: 5392-5402.

[507] Chung JY, Cho SJ and Hah JMi, A python-based docking program utilizing a receptor bound ligand shape:PythDock, Arch Pharm. Res, 2011, 34:1451-1458.

[508] Mashiach E, Schneidman-Duhovny D, Peri A, Shavit Y, Nussinov R and Wolfson HJ, An integrated suite of fast docking algorithms, Proteins, 2010, 78:3197-3204.

[509] Plewcznski D, Lazniewski M, Von Grothuss M, Rychiewski L, Ginalski K, VoteDock, Consensus docking method for prediction of protein-ligand interactions, J. Comput. Chem. 2011, 32: 568-581.

[510] Feng JA, Marshall GR, SKATE: A docking program that decouples systematic sampling from scoring, J. Comput. Chem. 2010, 31: 2540 - 2554

[511] Cabrera CA, Klett J, Dos Santos HG, Perona A, Gil-Redondo R, Francis SM, Priego EM, Gago F and Morreale A, J. CRDOCK: An ultrafast multipurpose Protein-Ligand Docking Tool. Chem. Information and Modeling, 2012, 52:2300-2309.

[512] Beato C, Beccari AR, Cavazzoni C, Lorenzi S and Constantino G, Use of experimental design to optimize docking performance: The case of ligenDock, the docking module of Ligen, a new *de Novo* design program, J. of Chemical Information and Modeling, 2013, 53: 1503-1517.

[513] Andrusier N, Nussinov R, Wolfson HJ, FireDock: Fast interaction refinement in molecular docking, Proteins, 2007, 69: 139-159.

[514] Takaya D, Yamashita A, Kamijo K, Gomi J, Ito M, Mackawa S, Enomoto N Sakamoto N, Watanabe Y, Arai R, Umeyama H, Honma T, Matsumoto T, Yokoyama S, A new method for induced fit docking (GENIUS) and its application to virtual screening of novel HCV NS3-4A protease inhibitors, Bioorganic and Medicinal Chemistry, Bioorganic and Medicinal Chemistry, 2011, 19: 6892-6905.

[515] Kim DS, Kim CM, Won CI, Kim JK, Ryu J, Cho Y, Lee C and Bhak J, BetaDock:Shape-priority docking method based on Beta-Complex, J. Biomolecular Structure and Dynamics, 2011, 29: 219-242.

[516] Meier R, Pippel M, Brandt F, Sippl W and Baldauf C, ParaDockS: A framework for molecular docking with population-based metaheuristics, J. Chem. Inf. Model, 2010, 50:879-889.

[517] Bullock C, Cornia n, Jacob R, Remm A, Peavey T, Weekes K, Mallory, Oxford JT, McDougal OM, Andersen TL, Dockomatic 2,0:High throughput inverse virtual screening and homology modeling, J Chem. Inf. Model. 2013, 53: 2161-2170.

[518] Ding F, Yin S and Dokholyan V, Rapid flexible docking using a stochastic rotamer library of ligands, J. Chem. Inf. Model, 2010, 50:1623-1632.

[519] Shin WH, Heo Lee J, Ko J, Seok C and Lee J, LigDockCSa:Protein-ligand docking using conformational space annealing, J. of Comp. Chem., 2011, 32: 3226-3232

[520] Vorobjev YN, Blind docking method combining search of low-resolution binding sites with ligand pose refinement by molecular dynamics-based global optimization, J. Comp. Chem. 2010, 31:1080-1092.

[521] Klenner A, Weisel M, Reisen F, Proschak E, Schneider G, Automated docking of flexible molecules into receptor binding sites by ligand self-organization *in situ*, Mol. Inf. 2010, 29:189-193.

[522] R Abagyan, M Totrov, D Kuznetsov. ICM—a new method for protein modeling and design:applications to docking and structure prediction from the distorted native conformation. J. Comp. Chem. 15, 5: 488-506.

[523] Ewing TJA, Makino S, Skillman AG and Kuntz ID, Dock4:0: Search strategies for automated molecular docking of flexible molecule databases, J. Computer-aided Molecular Design, 2001, 18:411-428.

[524] Liu M, Wang S, McDock; a Monte Carlo simulation approach to the molecular docking problem, J. of Computer-aided molecular design, 1999, 13: 435-451.

[525] Davis IW, Raha K, Head MS, Baker D, Blind Docking of pharmaceutically relevant compounds using Rosetta Ligand, Protein Science; 2008, 18:1998-2002.

[526] Brylinski M, Skolnich J, Q-DockLHM: Low-resolution refinement for ligand comparative modeling. J. Comput. Chem; 2010, 31:1093-1105.

[527] Liu HM, Huang HL, Hwang SF, Bo SY, SODOCK: Swarm optimization for highly flexible protein-ligand docking, J. Comput. Chem; 2007, 28: 612-623.

[528] Nikolic D, Blinov N, Wishart D and Kovalenko A, 3d-rism-dock: a new fragment-based drug design protocol, J. of Chemical Theory and Computation, 2012, 8: 3356-3372.

[529] Liu Y, Zhao L, Li W, Zhao D, Song M and Yang Y, FIPSDOCK: A new molecular docking technique driven by fully informed swarm optimization algorithm, J. of computational Chemistry, 2013, 34: 67-75.

[530] Thomsen R, Christensen MH, Moldock: a new technique for high-accuracy molecular docking. J. Med. Chem, 2006, 11:3315-3321.

[531] Kotasthane A, Mulakala C, Viswanadhan VM, Applying conformational selection theory to improve crossdocking efficiency in 3-phosphoinositide dependent protein kinase-1, Proteins, 2014:82:436-451.

[532] Ellingston SR, Smith JC and Baudry J, VinaMPI: Facilitating multiple receptor high-throughput virtual docking on high-performance computer, J. of Computational Chem, 2013, 34:2212-2221.

[533] Liu Chi, He G, Jiang Q, Han B and Peng C. Novel hybrid virtual screening protocol based on molecular docking and structure-based pharmacophore for discovery of methionyl-rRNA synthetase inhibitors as antibacterial agents, Int. J. Mol. Sci. 2013, 14: 14225-14239

[534] Balius TE, Allen WJ, Mukherjee S, Rizzo RC, Grid-based molecular footprint comparison method for docking and *de novo* design: Application to HIVgp41, J. of Comput. Chem, 2013:34:1226-1240.

[535] Therrien E, Englebienne P, Arrowsmith AG, Mendoza-Sanchez R, Corbeil CR, Weill N, Campagna-Slater V, Moitessier N, Integrating medicinal chemistry, organic/combinatorial chemistry and computational chemistry for the discovery of selective estrogen receptor modulators with Forecaster, a novel platform for drug Discovery, J. Chem. Inf. Model, 2012, 52: 210-224.

[536] Fang J, Huang D, Zhao W, Ge H, Luo HB and Xu J, A new protocol for predicting Novel GSK-3β ATP competitive inhibitors, Chem. Information and Modeling, 2011, 51: 1451-1438.

[537] Luo W, Pei J, Zhu Y, A fast protein-ligand docking alrithm based on hydrogen bond matching and surface shape complementarity, J. Mol. Model. 2010, 16: 903-913.

[538] Shin WH and Seok C, GalaxyDock:Protein-ligand docking with flexile protein sidechains, Chem. Inf. And Modeling, 2012, 52: 3225- 3232.

[539] Alisaraie L, Haller LA and Fels G, A QXP-based multistep docking procedure for accurate prediction of protein-ligand complexes, J. Chem. Info. Model, 2006, 46:1174-1187.

[540] Parenti MD, Rastelli G, Advances and applications of binding affinity prediction methods in durg discovery, Biotechnology Advances, Biotechnology Advances, 2012, 30:244-250.

[541] Antes I, DynaDock: A new molecular dynamics-based algorithm for protein-peptide docking including receptor flexibility, Proteins, 2010, 78:1084-1104.

[542] Okamato M, Masuda Y, Muroya A, Yasuno K, Takahashi O and Furuya T, Evaluation of docking calculation on X-ray structures using Consensus-Dock, Chem. Pharm Bull, 2010, 58: 1655 - 1657.

[543] Molecular Operating Environment (MOE), 2013.08; Chemical Computing Group Inc., 1010 Sherbooke St. West, Suite #910, Montreal, QC, Canada, H3A 2R7, 2013.

[544] Labute P, Williams C. Feher M, Sourial E, Schmidt JM. Flexible Alignment of Small Molecules; J. Med. Chem. 2001, 44: 1483-1490.

[545] Abad-Zapatero C, Chapter 8- Sightseeing Chemicobiological Space, In Ligand Efficiency Indices for Drug Discovery; Academic Press (2013) pp 109-149.546

[546] Molegro Virtual Docker 5.5 **(http://www.clcbio.com).**

[547] Muegge I and Martin YC. A general and fast scoring function for protein-ligand interactions J. Med. Chem. 1999, 42:791-804.

[548] Huang SY and Zou X. Inclusion of solvation and entropy in the knowled-based scoring functions for protein-ligand interactions. J. Chem. Inf. Model. 2010, 50: 262-273.

[549] Kroemer RT, Vulpetti A, McDonald JJ, Rohrer DC, Troset JY, Giordanetto F, Cotesta S, McMartin C, Kihlen M and Stouten PF. Assessment of docking poses: interactions-based accuracy classification (IBAC) *versus* crystal structure derivations. J. Chem. In. Comput. Sci. 2004, 44: 871-881.

[550] Yusuf D, Davis AM, Kleywegt GJ and Schmitt. An Alternative Method for the Evaluation of Docking Performance: RSR *vs*. RMSD. J. Chem. Inf. Model. 2008, 48: 1411-1422.

[551] Baber JC, Thompson J, Cross B and Humblet C. Modeling and active site refinement for G protein-coupled receptors J. Chem. Inf. Model. 2009, 49: 1889-1900.

[552] Jain AN. J. Modeling and active site refinement for G protein-coupled receptors. Comput-Aided Mol. Des. 2000, 14:199-213.

[553] Liu J, He X and Zhang JZH. Improving the scoring of protein-ligand binding affinity by including the effects of structural water and electronic polarization. Chemical information and modeling. 2013, 53, 1306−1314

[554] Wang W, He W, Zhou X and Chen X. Optimization of molecular docking scores with support vector rank regression. Proteins. 2013, 81:1386-1398.

[555] Alder BJ, Wainwright TE, Phase transition for a hard-sphere systemJ Chem. Phys. 1957, 27:1208

[556] Gibson JB, Goland AN, Miligrim M and Vineyard GH, Dynamics of radiation damage. Physics Rev.,1960, 120:1229.

[557]   Rahman AP. Correlations in the motion of atoms in liquid argon. Phys. Rev. 1964, 2A:405.

[558]   Holtje ED, Sippl W, Rognan D and Fulkers G. Molecular Modeling, Basic principles and Applications, 2003, 2n edition, Wiley-VCH, Darmstad.

[559]   Brooks BR, Bruccoleri RE, Olafson BD, States DJ, Swaminathan S and Karplus M. CHARMM:a program for macromolecular energy, minimization, and dynamics calculations Journal of Comp. Chem. 1983, 4: 187-217.

[560]   Hermans J, Berendsen HJC, Vangunsteren WF and Postma JPM, A consistent empirical potential for water-protein interactions Biopolymers, 1984, 25:1513.

[561]   Cornell WD, Cieplax P, Bayly CI, Gould IR, Merz KM, Ferguson DM, Spellmeyer DC, Fox T, Caldwell JW and Kollman PA. A Second Generation Force Field for the Simulation of. Proteins, Nucleic Acids, and Organic Molecules J. Am. Chem. Soc. 1995, 117:5179-5197.

[562]   Nelson MT, Humphrey W, Gursoy A, Dalke A, Kale LV, Skeel RD and Schulten K. NAMD:A parallel, object oriented molecular dynamics program International Journal Supercomputer Applications. 1996, 10:251.

[563]   Daubur-Osguthorpe P, Roberts VA, Osguthorpe DJ, Wolff J, Genesett M and Haggler AT. Structure and energetics of ligand binding to proteins: Escherichia coli dihydrofolate reductase-trimethoprim, a drug-receptor system Proteins: Functions, structure and Genes. 1988, 4:31

[564]   Hill TL, An introduction to statistical thermodynamics. 1960. An introduction to Statistical Thermodynamics. Addison-Wesley Publishing Company, New York.

[565]   Verlet L.Computer" experiments" on classical fluids. I. Thermodynamical properties of Lennard-Jones molecules Phys. Rev. 1967, 165: 201.

[566]   Beeman DJ. Some multistep methods for use in molecular dynamics calculations Comput. Phys. 1976, 20:130.

[567]   Hockney RW. The potential calculations and some application Methods Comput. Phys. 1970, 9:135-210.

[568]   Rykaert JP, Ciccotti G and Berendsen HJC. Numerical integration of cartesian equations of motion of a system with constraints- molecular dynamics of n-alkanes, J. Compt. Phys. 1977, 23:227.

[569]   Myamoto S and Kollman PA, SETTLE: an analytical version of the SHAKE and RATTLE algorithm for rigid water models J. Comput. Chem. 1992, 13:952-962.

[570]   Hess B and Bekker H, Berendsen HJC and Fraaije JGEM, LINCS: A linear constraint solver for molecular simulations J. Comp. Chem. 1997,18:1463-1472.

[571]   Lee SH, Palmo K and Krimm S. WIGGLE: A new constrained molecular dynamics algorithm in Cartesian coordinates J. Comp. Chem. 2005, 210:171-182.

[572]   Anderson HC, Rattle: A velocity version of the shake algorithm for molecular dynamics calculations J. Comp. Phys. 1983, 52:24-34.

[573]   Anderson HC. Molecular dynamics simulations at constant pressure and/or temperature J. Chem. Phys. 1980, 72:2384.

[574]   Berendsen HJC, Postma JPM, van Gunsteren WF, DiNola A and Haak JR. Molecular dynamics with coupling to an external bath J. Chem. Phys. 1984, 81:3684.

[575]   Nose S. A unified formulation of the constant-temperature molecular-dynamics methods J. Chem. Phys. 1984, 81:511.

[576]   Parinello M and Rahman A. Polymorphic transitions in single crystals: A new molecular dynamics method J. Appl. Phys. 1981, 52:7182.

[577] Shen J, Quiocho FA. Calculation of binding energy differences for receptor-ligand systems using the Poisson-Boltzmann method. J. Comp. Chem. 1995;16:445-453.

[578] Mullins E, Liu YA, Ghaderi A and Fast SD. Sigma Profile Database for predicting solid solubility in pure and mixed solvent mixtures for organic pharmacological compounds with cosmo-based thermodynamic methods. Ind. Eng. Chem. Res 2008;47:1707-1725

[579] Kollman PA, Massova I, Reyes C, Kuhn B, Huso OS, Chong L, Lee M, Lee T, Duan Y, Wang W, Donini AO, Cieplack, Srinivasan P, Case J, Cheatham TE. Calculating structures and free energies of complex molecules: combining molecular mechanics and continuum models. Acc. Chem. Res. 2000; 33:889-897.

[580] Shivakumar D, Deng Y and Roux B. Computations of absolute solvation free energies of small molecules using explicit and implicit solvent model. J. of Chem. Theory and Computation. 2009,5:919-930.

[581] Lerner MG, Meagher KL and Carlson HA. Automatied clustering of probe molecules from solvent mapping of protein surfaces: new algorithms applied to hot-spot mapping and structure-based drug design. J. Comput. Aided Mol. Des. 2008;22:727-736.

[582] Sun XM, Wei XG, Wu XP, Ren Y, Wong NB and Li WK. Cooperative effect of solvent in the neutral hydration of ketenimine: an *ab initio* study using the hybrid cluster/continuum model. J. Phys. Chem. A, 2010,114:595-602.

[583] Kosugi T, Nakanishi I and Kitaura K. Binding free energy calculations of adenosine deaminase inhibitor and the effect of methyl substitution in inhibitors. J. Chem. Inf. Model. 2009, 49: 615- 622.

[584] Knight JL and Brooks III CL. λ-dynamics free energy simulation methods J. Comput. Chem. 2009, 30:1692-1700.

[585] Kostjukov VV, Khomytova NM and Evstigneev MP. Partition of thermodynamic energies of Drug-DNA complexation. Biopolymers 2009, 91:773- 789.

[586] Mulakala C and Kaznessis YN. Path-integral method for predicting relative binding affinities of protein-ligand complexes. J. Am. Chem. Soc. 2009, 131: 4521-4528.

[587] Oostenbrink C. Efficient free energy calculations on small molecule host-guest systems - A combined linear interaction energy/one-step perturbation approach. J. Comput. Chem. 2009, 30: 212 -221.

[588] Nervall M, Hanspers P, Carlsson J, Boukharta L and Aqvist J. Predicting binding modes from free energy calculations. J. Med. Chem. 2008, 51:2657-2667.

[589] Cossins BP, Foucher S, Edge CM and Essex JW. Assessment of nonequilibrium free energy methods. J. Phys. Chem. B 2009, 113:5508-5519.

[590] Banavali NK, Im W, Roux B. Electrostastic free energy calculations using the generalized solvent boundary potential method. J. Chem. Phys. 2002, 117:7381-7388.

[591] Chipot C, Rozanska X, Dixit SB. Can free energy calculations be fast and accurate at the same time? Binding of low-affinity, nonpeptide inhibitors to the SH2 domain of the Src protein. J. Comput. Aided Mol. Des. 2005, 19:765-770.

[592] Jarzynski C. Nonequilibrium equality for free energy differences. Phys. Rev. Lett. 1997, 78:2690-2693.

[593] Shirts MR, Hooker EB and Pande VS. Equilibrium free energies from nonequilibrium measurements using maximum-likelihood methods. Phys. Rev. Lett. 2003, 91:140601-140604

[594] Suarez D, Diaz N and Lopez R. A combined semiempirical and DFT computational protocol for studying bioorganometallic complexes: application to molybdocene-cysteine complexes. J. Comp. Chem., 2014, 35;324-334.

[595] Mayn CG, Saam J, Schulten K, Tajkharshid E and Gunbart JC, Rapid parameterization of small molecules using the force field Tookit. J. Comput. Chem. 2013, 348: 2757-2770.

[596] Kara M and Zacharias M. Stabilization of duplex DNA and RNA by dangling ends studied by free energy simulations. Biopolymers, 2014, DOI 10.1002/bip.22398.

[597] Wang W; Wang J, Kollman PA. What determines the van der Waals coefficient β in the LIE (linear energy) method to estimate binding free energies using molecular dynamics simulations. Proteins 1999, 34:395-402.

[598] Shirts MR and Pande VS. Comparison of efficiency and bias of free energies computed by exponential averaging, the Bennett acceptance ratio and thermodynamic integration. The Journal of Chemical Physics 2005, 122:144107-144108.

[599] Zhou R, Friesner RA, Ghosh A, Rizzo RC, Jorgensen WL, Levy RM. New linear interaction mehod for binding affinity calculations using a continuum solvent model. J. Phys. Chem. B 2001, 105:10388-10397.

[600] Grater F, Schwarzl SM, Dejaegere A, Fischer S, Smith JC. 2005; Protein/ligand binding free energies calculated with quantum mechanics/molecular mechanics. J. Phys. Chem. B. 2005, 109:10474-10483.

[601] Wu D and Kofke DA. Phase-space overlap measures.I. Fail-safe bias detection in free energies calculated by molecular simulation. The Journal of Chemical Physics 2005, 54103-54110.

[602] Woods CJ and Essex JW. Enhanced configurational sampling in binding free-energy calculations. J. Phys. Chem. B 2003, 107:13711-13718.

[603] Woods CJ, Essex JW and King MA. The development of replica-exchange-based free-energy methods. J. Phys. Chem. B 2003, 107:13703-13710.

[[604] Foloppe N and Hubbard R. Towards predictive ligand design with free-energy based computational methods. Current medicinal chemistry. 2006, 13:3583-3608.

[605] Wu D and Kofke A. Rosenbluth-sampled nonequilibrium work method for calculation of free energies in molecular simulation. The Journal of Chemical Physics 2005, 122:204104-204113.

[606] loppe Pohorille A, Chipot C. Eds. Free energy calculatiohns-Theory and applications in chemistry and biology; Springer: Heidelberg, 2007.

[607] Kerrigan JE, Molecular dynamics simulations indrug design, *In silico* models for drug discovery methods in molecular biology, 2013, 993: 95-113.

[608] Zwanzig RW. High-temperature equation of state by a perturbation method. I. Nonpolar gases. J. Chem. Phys. 1954, 22:1420-1426.

[609] Beutler TC, Mark AE, van Schaik RC, Gerber PPR, van Gunsteren WF. Avoiding singularities and numerical instabilities in free energy calculations based on molecular simulations. Chem. Phys. Lett. 1994, 222:529-539.

[610] Áqvist J, Medina C, Samuelsson JE. A new method for predicting binding affinity in computer-aided drug design. Protein Eng. 1994, 7:385-391.

[611] Oostenbrink BC, Pitzera JW, Van Lipzig MMH, Meerman, JHN, van Gunsteren WF. Simulations of the estrogen receptor ligand-binding domain: Affinity of natural ligands and Xenoestrogens. J. Med. Chem. 2000, 43: 4594-4605.

[612] Oostenbrink C, van Gunsteren WF. Free energies of binding of polychlorinated biphenyls to the estrogen receptor from a single simulation. Proteins 2004, 54:237-246.

[613] Woods CJ, Manby FR and Mulholland AJ. An efficient method for the calculation of quantum mechanics/molecular mechanics free energies. The J. of Chem. Phys. 2008, 128:14109-14117.

[614] Kumar S, Payne PW, Vasquez M. J. Method for free-energy calculations using iterative techniques. J. Comput. Chem. 1996,17:1269-1275.

[615] Michel J, Verdonk ML and Essex JW. Protein-ligand complexes: Computation of the relative free energy of different scaffolds and binding modes. J. Chem. Theory and Computation. 2007, 3:1645-1655.

[616] Hansmann UHE. Parallel tempering algorithm for conformational studies of biological molecules. Chem. Phys. Lett. 1997, 281:140-150.

[617] Faloppe N, Hubbard R. Towards predictive Ligand design with free-energy based computational methods? Curr. Med. Chem. 2006, 13:3583-3608.

[618] Ashbaugh HS, Asthagiri D. Single ion hydration free energies: A consistent comparison between experiment and classical molecular simulation. J. Chem. Phys. 2008, 129: 204501-204506.

[619] Guo Z, Brooks CL III, Kong X. Efficient and flexible algorithm for free energy calculations using the λ-dynamics approach. J. Phys. Chem. B 1998, 102:2032-2036.

[620] Biletti-Putzer R, Yang W, Karplus M. Generalized ensembles serve to improve the convergence of free energy simulations. Chem. Phys. Lett. 2003, 377:693-641.

[621] Damodaran KV, Banba S, Brooks CL III. Application of multiple topology λ-dynamics to a host-guest system β-Cyclodextrin with substituted benzenes. J. Phys. Chem. B. 2001, 105:9316-9322.

[622] Banba S, Brooks CL III. Free energy screening of small ligands bindng to an artificial protein cavity. J. Chem. Phys. 2000, 113:3423-3433.

[623] Brooks BR, Bruccoleri RE, Olafson BD, Sates DJ, Swaminuthan S, Karplus M. CHARMM:a program for macromolecular energy, minimization and dynamics calculations J. Comp. Chem. 1983, 4:187-217.

[624] Pitera J, Kollman PA. Designing an optimum guest for a host using mutimolecule free energy calculations: Predicting the best. J. Am Chem. Soc. 1998, 120:7557-7567.

[625] Guo Z, Brooks CL III. Rapid screening of binding affinities:Application of the λ-dynamics method to a trypsin-inhibitor system. J. Am. Chem. Soc. 1998,120:1920-1921.

[626] Zoete V, Michielin O, Karplus M. Protein-ligand binding free energy estimation using molecular mechanics and continmuum electrostatics. Application to HIV-1 protease inhibitors. J. Comput.-Aided Mol. Des. 2003,17:861-880.

[627] Wu D, Kofke DA, Phase-space overlap measures. II. Design and implementation of staging methods for free-energy calculations. J. Chem. Phys. 2005,126293:84109-84110.

[628] Mobley DL, Graves AP, Chodera JD, McReynolds AC, Stoichet BK and Dill KA. Predicting absolute ligand binding free energies to a simple model site. J. Mol. Biol. 2007,371:1118-1134.

[629] Pearlman DA, Koffman PA. The lag between the Hamiltonian and the system configuration in free energy perturbation calculations. J. Chem. Phys. 1989, 91:7831-7839.

[630] Lee MS, Salsbury FR, Brooks CL. Constant-pH molecular dynamics using continuous titration coordinates. Proteins 2004;56:738-752.

[631] Abrams JB, Rosso L, Tuckerman ME. Efficient and precise solvation free energies *via* alchemical adiabatic molecular dynamics. J. Chem. Phys. 2006;125;74115-74127.

[632] Stock G, Jain A, Riccardi L, Nguyen PI, Conformational Analysis of Unfolded States. Exploring the Energy Landscape of Small Peptides and Proteins by Molecular Dynamics Simulations. Gerhard Stock, Abhinav Jain, Laura Riccardi, Phuong H Nguyen. Edited by

Schweitzer-Stenner- Reinhard, From Protein and Peptide Folding, Misfolding, and Non-Folding (2012), Pp 57-77. |

[633] Pitera JW, Kollman PA. Exhaustive mutagenesis *in silico*:multicoordinate free energy calculations on proteins and peptides. Proteins. 2000; 41;385-397.

[634] Real F, Vallet, V, Flament JP, Masella M, Revisiting a many-body model for water based on a single polarizable site: From gas phase clusters to liquid and air/liquid water systems. Journal of Chemical Physics. 2013, 139: 11-16.

[635] Zhou S, Solana JR. Monte Carlo and theoretical calculations of the first four perturbation coefficients in the high temperature series expansion of the free energy for discrete and core-softened potential models. J. Chem. Phys. 2013,139: 049901-0499011.

[636] Mahmut K, Martin Z. Stabilization of duplex DNA and RNA by dangling ends studied by free energy simulations. Biopolymers. 2014, 101: 4, 418-427.

[637] Benjamin R, Horbach J. Wall-liquid and wall-crystal interfacial free energies *via* thermodynamic integration: A molecular dynamics simulation study. J. Chem. Phys. 2012,137: 39901-39902.

[638] Banks D, Latypov RF. Ketchem RR, Woodard J, Scavezze JL, Siska CC, Razinkov V I. J. Pharm. Sci., 2012: 101, 2720-2732.

[639] Lee JY, Kang NS, Kang YK. Reply to "comment on binding free energies of inhibitors to iron porphyrin complex as a model for cytochrome P450 Biopolymers, 2012, 97: 649-650.

[640] Kopitz H, Cashman DA, Pfeiffer-Marek S, Gohlke H. Influence of the solvent representation on vibrational entropy calculations: Generalized born *versus* distance-dependent dielectric model. Journal of Computational Chemistry.2012, 33:1004-1013.

[641] Rydberg P. Binding free energies of inhibitors to iron porphyrin complex as a model for cytochrome p450. Comment. Biopolymers. 2012, 97: 250-251.

[642] Limmer DT, Chandler D, The putative liquid-liquid transition is a liquid-solid transition in atomistic models of water. II. Journal of Chemical Physics. 2013, 138:21: 1-15

643] By Mobley, David L.; Liu, Shaui; Cerutti, David S.; Swope, William C.; Rice, Julia E. Testing the semi-explicit assembly solvation model in the SAMPL3 community blind test. Journal of Computer-Aided Molecular Design 2012, 26: 563-568

[644] Li YHC, Jing-Zhen L, Xue-Mei ZL. Multiphase equation of states of the solid and liquid phases of Al and Ta. Chinese Physics Letters 2012, 29:1-4.

[645] Malhado JP, Spezia R, Hynes JT. Conical intersection structure and dynamics for a model protonated schiff base photoisomerization in solution. International Journal of Quantum Chemistry 2013, 16: 7.

[646] Da Silva JCS, Rocha WR. C-H bond activation of methane in aqueous solution: A hybrid quantum mechanical/effective fragment potential study. J. Comp. Chem. 2011, 32: 3383-3392.

[647] Du J, Sun H, Xi, L, Li J, Yang Y, Liu H, Yao X. Molecular modeling study of checkpoint kinase 1 inhibitors by multiple docking strategies and prime/MM-GBSA calculation. Journal of Computational Chemistry. 2011, 32: 2800-2820.

[648] Steiner D, Oostenbrink C, Diederich F, Zuercher M, van Gunsteren WF. Calculation of binding free energies of inhibitors to plasmepsin II. J. Comp. Chem. 2011: 32: 1801-1812.

[649] Kehoe CW, Fennell CJ. Dill KA. Testing the semi-explicit assembly solvation model in the SAMPL3 community blind test J. comp.-aided mol. design. 2012, 26: 563-568.

[650] Mobley DL; Liu S, Cerutti DS; Swope WC; Rice JE. Alchemical prediction of hydration free energies for SAMPL Journal of computer-aided molecular design 2012, 26: 551-562.

[651] Dubey KD, Tiwari RK, Ojha RP. Recent Advances in Protein-Ligand Interactions: Molecular Dynamics Simulations and Binding Free Energy. Current Computer-Aided Drug Design. 2013, 9: 518-531.

[652] Florent Réal, Valérie Vallet, Jean-Pierre Flament and Michel Masella, Revisiting a many-body model for water based on a single polarizable site: From gas phase clusters to liquid and air/liquid water systems. J. Chem. Phys. 2013, 139, 114502;

[653] Ghosh S, Ghosh SK. Density functional theory of surface tension of real fluids using a double well type Helmholtz free energy functional: application to water and heavy water. Molecular Physics. 2013, 111: 589-593.

[654] Cavalli A, Carloni P and Recanatini M. Tartet-related applications of first principles Quantum Chemical Methods in Drug Design. Chemical Reviews. 2006;106:3497-3519.

[655] Seifert G, Joswig JO. From Wiley Interdisciplinary Reviews: Computational Molecular Science, 2012, 2: 456-465.

[656] Gaus M, Cui Q, Elstner M, Wiley Interdisciplinary Reviews: Computational Molecular Science. 2014, 4: 49-61.

[657] Michael G, Qiang C and Marcus E. Density functional tight binding: application to organic and biological molecules. Interdisciplinary Reviews: Computational Molecular Science. 2014, 4: 49-61.

[658] Warshel A. Computer simulations of enzyme catalysis: Methods, progress and insights. Annu. Rev. Biophys. Biomol. Struct. 2003, 32:425-443.

[659] Car R, Parinello M. Unified approach for molecular dynamics and density-functional theory. Phys. Rev. Lett. 1985, 55:2471-2474.

[660] Waller MP, Robertazzi A, Plats JA, Hibbs DE, Williams PA. Hybrid densitgy functional theory for π-stacking interactions:Application to benzenes, pyridines and DNA bases. J. Comput. Chem. 2006, 27:491-504.

[661] Hohenberg P, Kohn W. Inhomogeneous electron gas. Physical Review B 1964;136:864-871.; Kohn W, Sham L. Self-consistent equations including exchange and correlation effects. J. Phys. Rev. A 1965, 149:1133-1138.

[662] Dans PD and Coitiño, Density functional theory characterization and descriptive analysis of cisplatin and related compounds. J. Chem. Inf. Model. 2009, 49:1407-1419.

[663] Guadarrama P, Soto-Castro D and Otero JR. Performance of DFT hybrid functional in the theoretical treatment of H-bonds:Analysis term-by-term. International Journal of Quantum Chemistry 2007, 108:229-237.

[[664] Koch W, Holthausen MC. A Chemist's Guide to density functional theory: Wiley-VCH; Weinheim, Germany 2000.

[665] Parr RG, Yang W. Density functional theory of the electronic structure of molecules. Annu. Rev. Phys. Chem. 1995, 46:701-728.

[666] Parr RG, Yang W. Density-functional theory of atoms and molecules. Oxford University Press: Oxford, UD, 1989.

[667] Scuseria GE, Staroverov VN. In Theory and applications of computational chemistry: The first forty years; Dykstra CE, Frenking G, Kim KS, Scuseria GE, Eds. Elsevier :Amsterdam; 2005.

[668] de Proft F, Sablon N, Tozer DJ, Geerlings P. Calculation of negative electron affinity and aqueous anion hardness using Kohn-Sham HOMO and LUMO energies. Faraday Discuss. 2007, 135:151-159.

[669] Becke AD. Density-functional thermochemistry. III. The role of exact exchange. J. Chem. Phys. 1993, 98:5648-5652.

[670] Schwabe T, Grimme S. Phys. Chem. Chem. Phys. Double-hybrid density functional with long-range dispersion correctitons:higher accuracy and extended applicability. 2007, 9:3397-3406.

[671] Van Caillie C, Amos RD. Geometric derivatives of excitation energies using SCF and DFT. Chem. Phys. Lett. 1999, 308:249-255.

[672] Scalmani G, Frisch MJ, Mennucci B, T omasi J, Cammi R, Barone V. Geometries and properties of excited states in the gas phase and in solution: Theory and application of a time-dependent density functional theory polarizable continuum model. J. Chem. Phys. 2006, 124, 94107-94122.

[673] Grimme S, Steinmetz M, Korth M. How to compute isomerization energies of organic molecules with quantum chemical methods. J. Org. Chem. 2007, 72:2118-2126.

[674] Schreiner PR. Angew. Chem. Int. Ed. Relative energy computations with approximate density functional theory- A caveat. Chem. Int. Ed. 2007, 46:4217-4219.

[675] Polo V, Grafenstein J, Krala E, Cremer D. Long-range and short-range Coulomb correlation effects as simulated by Hartree-Fock, local density approximation, and generalized gradient approximation exchange functional. Theor. Chem. Acc. 2003:109:22-35.

[676] Handy NC, Cohen AJ. Left-right correlation energy. Mol. Phys. 2001, 99:403-412.

[677] Xu X, Zhong Q, Muller RP, Goddard WA, III. An extended hybrid density functional (X3LYP) with improved descriptions of nonbond interactions and thermodynamic properties of molecular systemsJ. Chem. Phys. 2005, 122:14105-14129.

[678] Perdew JP, Burke K, Ernzerhof M. Phys. Generalized Gradient Approximation Made Simple. Phys. Rev. Lett. 1996,77:3865-3868.

[679] Quintal MM, Karton A, Iron MA, Boese AD, Martin JML. Benchmark Study of DFT Functionals for Late-Transition-Metal Reactions. J. Phys. Chem. A 2006, 110:709-716.

[680] Boese AD, Martin JML. Development of density functional for thermochemical kinetics. J. Chem. Phys. 2004, 121:3405-3416.

[681] Schirmer J, Dreuw A. Critique of the foundations of time-dependent density-functional theory. Phys. Rev A. 2007, 75:22513-22529.

[682] Dreuw A, Head-Gordon M. Single-Reference *ab Initio* Methods for the Calculation of Excited States of large Molecules Chem. Rev. 2005, 105:4009-4037.

[683] Sancho-Garcia JC. Assessing a new nonempirical density functional. J.Chem. Phys. 2006, 124:124112-12422

[684] Marques MAL, Gross EKU. The electron gas in TDDFT and SCDT. Annu. Rev. Phys. Chem. 2004, 55:427-455.

[685] Vydrov OA, Scuseria GE. Assessment of a long-range corrected hybrid functional. J. Chem. Phys. 2006, 125:234109-234118

[686] Furche F, Perdew JP. The performance of semilocal and hybrid density functionals in 3d transiion-metal chemistry. J. Chem. Phys. 2006, 124:44103-44130.

[687] Zhao Y and Truhlar DG. Density functionals with broad applicability in chemistry. Acc. Chem. Res 2008, 41:157-167.

[688] Tirado-Rives J, Jorgensen WL Performance of B3LYP density functional methods for a large set of organic molecules. J. Chem. Theor. Commun. 2008, 4:297-306.

[689] Hao MH. Theoretical calculation of hydrogen-bonding strength for drug molecules. J. of Chem. Theory and Computation. 2006, 2:363-872.

[690] Bouteiller Y, Poully JC, Desfrancois C and Gregoire G. Evaluation of MP2, DFT and DFT-D methods for the prediction of infrared spectra of peptides. J. Phys. Chem. A 2009, 113:6301-6307.

[691] Minenkov Y, Occhipinti G and Jensen VR. Metal-phosphine bond strengths of the transition metals: A challenge for DFT. J. Phys. Chem. A;2009, 113:11833-11844

[692] Wang YG. Examination of DFT and TDDFT Methods II. J. Phys. Chem. A 2009, 113:10873-10879.

[693] Scuseria GE, Staroverov VN. Progress in the development of exchange-correlation functionals. In Theory and application of computational chemistry: The first 40 years. Dykstra CE, Frenking G, Kim KS, Scuseria GE, EDs, Elsevier:Amsterdam, 2005.

[694] Y, Truhlar DG. The MO6 suite of densiy functionals for main group thermochemistry, thermochemical kinetics, noncovalent interactions, excited states and transition elements. Theor Chem. Acc. 2008, 120:215-241.

[695] Zhao Y, Schultz NE, Truhlar DG. Design of density functionals by combining the method of constraint satisfaction with parameterization for thermochemistry, thermochemical kinetics and noncovalent interactions. J. Chem. Theory Comput. 2006, 2:364-382.

[696] Mori-Sanchez P, Cohen AJ, Yan W. Many-electron self-interaction error in approximate density functionals. J. Chm. Phys. 2006,124:91102-91104.

[697] Perdew JP, Ruzsinsky A, Tão J, Staroverov VN, Scuseria GE, Csonka GI. Prescriptor for the design and selection of density functional approximations. J. Chem. Phys. 2005, 123, 62201-62209.

[698] Xu X, Goddard WA. The X3LYP extended functional to acurate decriptions of nonbonding interactions, spin states and thermochemical properties. Proc. Ntl. Acad. Sci. USA; 2004, 101:2673-2677.

[699] Grimme S. Semiempirical GGA-type densityy functional constructed with a long-range dispersion correction. J. Comput. Chem. 2006,27:1787-1799.

[700] Sato TA, Tsuneda T, Hirao K. A density-functional study on π-aromatic interactions. J. Chem. Phys 2005,123:104307-1043010.

[701] Jurecka P, Ceerny J. Hotza P, Salahub DR. DFT augmented with an empirical dispersion term. J. Comput. Chem. 2007, 28:555-569.

[702] Check CE, Gilbert TM. Progressive systematic underestimation of reaction energies in the B3LYP model as the number of C-C bonds increases. J. Org. Chem. 2005,60:9828-9834.

[703] Zhao Y, Truhlar DG. A density functional that accounts for medium-range correlation energies in organic chemistry. Org. Lett. 2006,8:5653-5756.

[704] Woodrich MD, Corminbouef C, Schreiner PR, Fokin AA and Schleyer PVR. How accurate are DFT treatments of organic energies? Org. Lett. 2007, 9:1851-1854.

[705] Schultz N, Zhao Y, Truhlar DG. Dnsity functional for inorganometallic and organometallic chemistry. J. Phys. Chem. A 2005, 109:11127-11143.

[706] Harvey JN. On the accuracy of DFT in transition metal chemistry. Annu. Rep. Prog. Chem. Sct 2006,104:4811-4 815.

[707] Zhao Y and Truhlar DG. Design of density functionals that are broadly accurate for hermochemistry, thermochemical kinetics and nonbonding interactions. J. Phys. Chem. A 2005, 109:5656 - 5667.

[708] Zhao Y, Truhlar DG. How well can new-generation density functionals methods describe stacking interactions in biological systems. Phys. Chem. Chem. Phys. 2005, 8:2701-2705.

[709] Zhao Y, Tishchenko O, Truhlar DG. How well can density functional methods describe hydrogen bonds to π acceptors? J. Phys. Chem. B 2005,109:19046-19051.

[710] Hamprecht FA, Cohen AJ, Tozer DJ, Handy NC. Development and assessment of new exchange-correlation functional. J. Chem. Phys. 1998, 199:6264-6271 [503].

[711] Kobayashi R, Amos RD. The application of CAM-B3lyp to the charge-transfer band problem of the zinc-bacteriochlorin complex. Chem. Phys. Lett. 2006, 420:106-109.

[712] Thonhauser T, Cooper VR, Li S, Puzder A, Hyldguard P, Langreth DC. Van der Waals density functional: Self-consistent potential and the nature of the van der Waals bond. Phys. Rev. B 2007,74:125112-125123.

[713] Pastor M, Cruciani G, Mclay I, Pickett S, Clementi S. GRid-INdependent descriptors (GRIND): a novel class of alignment- independent three-dimensional molecular descriptors. J. Med. Chem. 2000, 43: 3233-3243.

[714] Goodford PJ. A computational procedure for determining energetically favorable binding sites on biologically important macromolecules.506 J. Med. Chem. 1995, 28: 849-857.

[715] Duran A, Martinez GC, Pastor M. Development and Validation of AMANDA, a New Algorithm for Selecting Highly Relevant Regions in Molecular Interaction Fields. J. Chem. Inf. Model. 2008, 48: 1813-1823.

[716] Mor M, Rivara S, Lodola A, Lorenzi S, Bordi F, Plazzi PV, Spadoni G, Bedini A, Duranti A, Tontini A, Tarzia G. Application of 3D-QSAR in the rational design of receptor ligands and enzyme inhibitors. Chem. Biodivers. 2005, 2: 1438-1451.

[717] Mittal RR, Mckinnon RA, Sorich MJ. Effect of steric molecular field settings on CoMFA predictivity. J. Mol. Model. 2008, 14: 59-67.

[718] Klebe G, Abraham U, Mietzner T. Molecular similarity indexes in a comparative-analysis (CoMSIA) of drug molecules to correlate and predict their biological-activity. J. Med. Chem. 1994, 37: 4130-4146.

[719] Suh ME, Park SY, Lee HJ. Three-Dimensional QSAR Using the k-Nearest Neighbor Method and Its Interpretation. Bull. Korean Chem. Soc. 2002, 23: 417-422.

[720] Ul-Haq, Z., Wadood, A., Uddin, R., CoMFA and CoMSIA 3D-QSAR analysis on hydroxamic acid derivatives as urease inhibitors. 2009. J. Enz. Inhib. Med. Chem., 24, 272-278.

[721] Yang XS, Wang XD, Ji L, Li R, Sun C, Wang LS. Combining docking and comparative molecular similarity indices analysis (COMSIA) to predict estrogen activity and probe molecular mechanisms of estrogen activity for estrogen compounds. Chinese Sci Bull. 2008, 53: 3626-3633.

[722] Cruciani G; 2006. Molecular Interaction Fields: Applications in Drug Discovery and ADME Prediction, WILEY-VCH, Weinheim.

[723] Kastenholz MA, Pastor M, Cruciani G, Haaksma EEJ, Fox T. GRID/CPCA: A New Computational Tool to Design Selective Ligands. J. Med. Chem. 2000, 43: 3033-3044.

[724] Laurie ATR, Jackson RM. Q-SiteFinder: an energy-based method for the prediction of protein-ligand binding sites. Struct. Bioinf. 2005, 21: 1908-1916.

[725] Afzelius L, Masimirembwa CM, Karlén A, Andersson TB, Zamora I. Discriminant and quantitative PLS analysis of competitive CYP2C9 inhibitors *versus* non-inhibitors using alignment independent GRIND descriptors. J. Computer-Aided Mol. Design. 2002, 16: 433-458.

[726] Carosati E, Lemoine H, Spogli R, Grittner D, Mannhold R, Tabarrini O, Sabatini S, Cecche] tti V. Binding studies and GRIND/ALMOND-based 3D QSAR analysis of benzothiazine type K(ATP)-channel openers. Bioorg. Med. Chem. 2005, 13:5581-5591.

[727] Benedetti P, Mannhold R, Cruciani G, Ottaviani G. GRIND/ALMOND investigations on CysLT(1) receptor antagonists of the quinolinyl(bridged)aryl type. Bioorg. Med. Chem. 2004, 12: 3607-3617.

[728] Sciabola S, Carosati E, Baroni M, Mannhold R. Comparison of Ligand-Based and Structure-Based 3D-QSAR: A Case Study on (Aryl-)Bridged 2-Aminobenzonitriles Inhibiting HIV-1 Reverse Transcriptase. J. Med. Chem. 2005, 48: 3756-3767.

[729] Cianchetta G, Singleton RW, Zhang M, Wildgoose M, Giesing D, Fravolini A, Cruciani G, Vaz RJ. A pharmacophore hypothesis for P-glycoprotein substrate recognition using GRIND-based 3D-QSAR. J. Med. Chem. 2005, 48: 2927-2935.

[730] Fontaine F, Pastor M, Zamora I, Sanz F. Anchor-GRIND: Filling the gap between standard 3D-QSAR and the GRid-INdependent Descriptors. J. Med. Chem. 2005, 48: 2687-2694.

[731] Li Q, Jørgensen FS, Oprea T, Brunak S, Taboureau O. hERG classification model based on a combination of support vector machine method and GRIND descriptors. Mol. Pharm. 2008, 5: 117-127.

[732] Vyas V, Jain A, Jain A, Gupta A. Virtual Screening: A Fast Tool for Drug Design. Sci Pharm. 2008, 76: 333-360.

[733] Ahlstrm MM, Ridderstrm M, Luthman K, Zamora I. Virtual Screening and Scaffold Hopping Based on GRID Molecular Interaction Fields. J. Chem. Inf. Model. 2005, 45: 1313-1323.

[734] Schneider G, Böhm H. Virtual screening and fast automated docking methods. Drug Discov. Today. 2002,7:64-70.

[735] Neves MAC, Dinis TCP, Colombo G, Sa ML, Fast M. Fast Three Dimensional Pharmacophore Virtual Screening of New Potent Non-Steroid Aromatase Inhibitors J. Med. Chem. 2009, 52: 143-150.

[736] Wolohan PRN, Clark RD. Predicting drug pharmacokinetic properties using molecular interaction fields and SIMCA. J. Computer-Aided Mol. Design 2003,17: 65-76.

[737] MODI S. Computational approaches to the understanding of ADMET properties and problems. Drug Discov. Today. 2003, 8: 621-623.

[738]] O'Brien SE, Groot MJ. Greater than the sum of its parts: combining models for useful ADMET prediction. J. Med. Chem. 2005, 48: 1287-1291.

[739] Cruciani G., Pastor M, Guba W. VolSurf: a new tool for the pharmacokonetic optimization of lead compounds. Eur. J. Pharm. Sci. 2000, 2: S29-S39.

[740] Cruciani G, Crivori P, Carrupt PA, Testa B. Cruciani G, Crivori P, Carrupt PA, Testa B. J. Mol. Struct., 503, 17. 2000. J. Mol. Struct. 2000, 503: 17-30.

[741] Doddareddy MR, Cho YS, Koh HY, Kim DH, Pae AN. *In silico* renal clearance model using classical Volsurf approach. J. Chem. Inf. Model. 2006, 46: 1312-1320.

[742] Van de Waterbeemd H, Lennernäs H, Artursson P. Drug Bioavailability: Estimation of Solubility, Permeability, Absorption and Bioavailability, 2003; WILEY-VCH, Weinheim.

[743] Milletti F, Storchi L, Sforna G, Cruciani G, New and Original pK_a Prediction Method Using Grid Molecular Interaction Fields. J. Chem. Inf. Model. 2007, 47: 2172-2181.

[744] Sciabola S, Stanton RV, Mills JE, Floco MM, Baroni M, Cruciani G, Perrucio F and Mason JS. High-throughput virtual screening of proteins using GRID molecular interaction fields. Bioinformatics 2009, 25:3185-3200.

[745] Baroni M, Cruciani G, Sciabola S, Perruccio F and Mason JS. A common referene framework for analyzing/comparing proteins and ligand. Fingerprints for ligands and proteins (FLAP);Theory and application. J. Chem. Inf. Model. 2007, 47:279-294.

[746] Weisel M, Proschak E, Schneider G. PocketPicker:analysis of ligand binding-sites with shape descriptors. Chem. Cent. J. 2007, 1:1-17.

[747] GRID V.17:Molecular Discovery Ltd. West Way House. Elms Parade. Oxford. 1999.

[748]ALMOND v.2.0: Multivariate Infometric Analysis S.R.1. Viale del Castagni. 16.Perugia 2000.

[749] Ghersi D and Sanchez R. EasyMIFs and SiteHOUND: a tookit for the identification of ligand-binding sites in protein structures. Structural bioinformatics. 2009, 23:3185-3186.

[750] Huang J, Deng R, Wang J, Wu H, Xiong Y and Wang X, metaPIS A sequence-based Meta-server for protein interaction Site prediction, Protein & peptide letters, 2013, 20: 218-230.

[751] Berman HM, Westbrook J, Feng Z, Gilliland G, Bhat TN, *et al.* The protein data bank. Nucleic Acids Res 2000, 28: 235-42.

[752] Katchalski-Katzir E, Shariv I, Eisenstein M, Friesem AA, Aalo C, *et al.* Molecular surface recognition: determination of geometric fit between proteins and their ligands by correlation techniques. Proceedings of the National Academy of Sciences of the United States of America. 1992, 89: 2195-2199.

[753] Gabb HA, Jackson RM, Sternberg MJE, Modeling protein docking using shape complementarity, electrostatics and biochemical information. Journal of Molecular Biology, 1997, 272: 106-120.

[754] Ritchie DW, Kemp GJ. Protein docking using spherical polar Fourier correlations. Proteins: Structure, Function, and Genetics. 2000, 39: 178-194.

[755] Ritchie DW Parametric Protein Shape Recognition. Phd thesis, Departments of Computer Science & Molecular and Cell Biology, 1988. University of Aberdeen, King's College, Aberdeen, UK.

[756] Max NL, Getzoff ED. Spherical harmonic molecular surfaces. IEEE Computer Graphics & Applications. 1988, 8: 42-50.

[757] Kovacs JA, Chacon P, Cong Y, Metwally E, Wriggers W (2003) Fast rotational matching of rigid bodies by fast fourier transform acceleration of five degrees of freedom. Acta Crystallographica, Biological Crystallography D59: 1371-1376.

[758] Das R, Andre I, Shen Y, Wu Y, Lemak A, *et al.* Simultaneous prediction of protein folding and docking at high resolution. Proceedings of the National Academy of Sciences of the United States of America. 2009, 106: 18978-18983.

[759] Dominguez C, Boelens R, Bonvin AMJJ. Haddock: a protein-protein docking approach based on biochemical or biophysical information. Journal of the American Chemical Society.2003, 125: 1731-1737.

[760] Huang W, Liu H. Optimized grid-based protein-protein docking as a global search tool followed by incorporating experimentally derivable restraints. Proteins. 2012, 80: 691-702.

[761] Chen R, Weng Z. A novel shape complementarity scoring function for protein-protein docking. Proteins: Structure, Function, and Genetics. 2003, 51: 397-408

[762] Gu S, Koehl P, Hass J, Amenta N (2012) Surface-histogram: A new shape descriptor for protein-protein docking. Proteins: Structure, Function, and Bioinformatics.2012, 80: 221-238.

[763] Mandell JG, Roberts VA, Pique ME, Kotlovyi V, Mitchell JC, *et al.* (2001) Protein docking using continuum electrostatics and geometric fit. Protein Engineering 14: 105-113.

[764] Chen R, Weng Z.Docking unbound proteins using shape complementarity, desolvation, and electrostatics. Proteins: Structure, Function, and Genetics. 2002, 47: 281-294.

[765] Kozakov D, Brenke R, Comeau S, Vajda S. PIPER: An FFT-based protein docking program with pairwise potentials. Proteins: Structure, Function, and Bioinformatics.2006, 65: 392-406.

[766] Wright JD, Sargsyan, Wu X, Brooks BR, Lim C. Protein-protein docking using EMAP in CHARMM and support vector machine: Application to Ab/Ag complexes. J. Chem. Theor. Comput. 2013, 9:4186-4194.

[767] Ben-Zeev E, Berchanski A, Heifetz A, Shapira B, Eisenstein M. Prediction of the unknown: Inspiring experience with the CAPRI experiment. Proteins:Structure, Function, and Bioinfor- matics.2003 52: 41-46.

[768] Li L, Chen R, Weng Z. Rdock: Refinement of rigid-body protein docking predictions. Proteins: Structure, Function, and Genetics. 2003, 53: 693-707.

[769] Mintseris J, Pierce B, Wiehe K, Anderson R, Chen R, *et al.* Integrating statistical pair potentials into protein complex prediction. Proteins: Structure, Function, and Bioinformatics.2007, 69: 511-520.

[770] Garzon J, Lopez-Blanco J, Pons C, Kovacs J, Abagyan R, *et al.* FRODOCK: a new approach for fast rotational protein-protein docking. Bioinformatics. 2009, 25: 2544-2551.

[771] Ravikant DVS, Elber R. Pie - efficient filters and coarse grained potentials for unbound protein-protein docking. Proteins.2010, 78: 400-419.

[772] Liu S, Vakser IA. DECK: Distance and environment-dependent, coarse-grained, knowledge- based potentials for protein-protein docking. 2011, BMC Bioinformatics 12.

[773] Ritchie D W. Recent progress and future directions in protein-protein docking. Current protein and peptide Science, 2008, 9: 1-15.

[774] Chang-Seng Z, Lua-Hua L, Protein-Protein interactions, prediction, design and modulation. Acta Phys. Chem. Sim. 2012, 28: 2363-2380.

[775] Gray J. High-resolution protein-protein docking. Current opinion in structural biology. 2006, 16: 183-193.

[776] Bonvin A. Flexible protein-protein docking. Current opinion in structural biology. 2006, 16: 194-200.

[777] Halperin I, Ma B, Wolfson H, Nussinov R. Principles of docking: na overview of search algorithms and a guide to scoring functions. Proteins: Structure, Function, and bioinformatics. 2002, 47: 409-443.

[778] Castrillon-Candas J, Siddavanahalli V, Bajaj C. Nonequispaced Fourier ransforms for protein-protein docking. ICES Report. 2005,05-44, The University of Texas at Austin.

[779] Bajaj C, Chowdhury RA, Siddavanahalli V. F2Dock: Fast Fourier Protein-Protein Docking. IEEE/ACM Transactions on Computational Biology and Bioinformatics. 2011, 8: 45-58.

[780] Chowdhury RA, Bajaj C. Algorithms for faster molecular energetics, forces and interfaces. ICES report. 2010, 10-32, Institute for Computational Engineering & Science, The University of Texas at Austin.

[781] Bajaj C, Chowdhury RA, Rasheed M. A dynamic data structure for flexible molecular maintenance and informatics. Bioinformatics. 2010, 27: 55-62.

[782] Bajaj C, ZhaoW. Fast molecular solvation energetics and forces computation. SIAM Journal on Scientific Computing. 2010, 31: 4524-4552.

[783] Bajaj C, Djeu P, Siddavanahalli V, Thane A. TexMol: Interactive visual exploration of large flexible multi-component molecular complexes. In: Proc. Of the Annual IEEE Visualization Conference. 2004, pp. 243-250.

[784]   Mintseris J, Wiehe K, Pierce B, Anderson R, Chen R, *et al*. Protein-protein docking bench-mark 2.0: an update. Proteins. 2003, 60: 214-6.

[785]   Hwang H, Vreven T, Janin J, Weng Z.Protein-protein docking benchmark version 4.0. Proteins: Structure, Function, and Bioinformatics. 2010, 20178:3111-3114.

[786]   Mitchell JC. Sampling rotation groups by successive orthogonal images. SIAM Journal on Scientific Computing. 2008, 30: 525-547.

[787]   Bienstock RJ. Computational Drug design targeting Protein-Protein interactions. Current pharmaceutical drugs, 2012, 18: 1240-1254.

[788]   Chowdhury R, Rasheed M, Keidel D, Moussalem M, Olson A, Sanner M, Bajaj C. Protein-Protein Docking with F2Dock 2.0 and GB-Rerank. PlosOne. 2013, 51307:1-17.

[789]   Van Arnam EB and Dougherty DA, Functional probes of drug-receptor interactions implicated by structural studies:Cys-Loop receptors provide a fertile testing ground. J. Med. Chem. 2014, DOI: 10,1021/jm500023m.

[790]   Benighaus T, DiStasio RA, Lochan RC, Chai JD, Head-Gordon M. Semiempirical Double-Hybrid Density functional with improved description of long-range correlation. J. Phys. Chem A. 2008;112:2702-2712.

[791]   Tsuzuki S, Uchimaru T and Mikami M. Magnitude and nature of carbohydrate-aromatic interactions: *ab initio* calculations of fucose-benzene complex. J. Physics. Chem. B. 2009;113: 5617-5621

[792]   Hernandes MZ, Ponts FJ, Coelho LCD, Moreira DRM, Pereira VRA and Leite ACL. Recent insights on the medicinal chemistry of metal-based compounds:Hints for the successful drug design, Current Medicinal Chemistry, 2010, 17: 3739-3750.

[793]   Hagiwara Y and Tateno M. A novel computational scheme for acurate and efficient evaluation of π stacking. J. Phys Condens. Matt. 2009,21:245103-245108.

[794]   Waller MP, Robertazzi A, Plats JA, Hibbs DE, Williams PA. Hybrid densitgy functional theory for π-stacking interactions:Application to benzenes, pyridines and DNA bases. J. Comput. Chem. 2006, 27:491-504.

[795]   Benighaus T, DiStasio RA, Lochan RC, Chai JD, Head-Gordon M. Semiempirical Double-Hybrid Density functional with improved description of long-range correlation. J. Phys. Chem A. 2008,112:2702-2712.

[796]   Hatty CR, Le Brun AP, Lake V, Clifton LA, Liu GJ, James M, Banati R. Investigating the interactions of the 18 kDa translocator protein and its ligand PK11195 in planar lipid bilayers. BBA-Biomembranes, 2014, 1838:1019-1030.

[797]   Hu G, Kuang G, Xiao W, Li W, Li G, Tang Y Performance evaluation of 2D fingerprint and 3D shape similarity methods in virtual screening. J Chem. Inf. Model. 2012, 52: 1103-1113.

[798]   Planesas J, Claramunt RM,Texido J, Borell Jl, Perez-Nueno VI, Improving VEGFR-2 docking-based screening by pharmacophore postfiltering and similarity search postprocessing. J. Chem. Inf. Model. 2011, 31: 777-787.

[799]   Eckert H, Bajorah J. Molcular similarity analysis in virtual screening: foundations, limitations and novel approaches. *Drug Discovery Today*. 2007, 12:225-253.

[800]   Lingenfelder M *et al*. Tracking the chiral recognition of of adsorbed dipeptides at the single-molecule level. *Angew. Chem. Int. Ed. English*. 2007, 46:4492-4495.

[801]   Ballester PJ and Richards WG. Ultrafast shape recognition to search compound databases for similar molecular shapes. J. Comp. Chem. 2007, 28: 1711-1723.

[802] Wells JA, McClendon CL. Reaching for high-hanging fruit in drug discovery at protein-protein interfaces. Nature 2007, 450: 1001-1009.

[803] Brey DM *et al.* High-throughput screening of a small molecule library for promoters and inhibitors of mesenchymal of stem cell osteogenic differentiation. Biotechnol. Bioeng. 2011, 108: 163-174.

[804] Ramachandran PV, Focusing on boron in medicinal chemistry. Future medicinal chemistry. 2013, 5:611-612.

[805] Chen W, Enck S, RICE jl, Powers DL, Powers ET, Wong CH, Dyson HJ and Kely JW. Strctural and energetic basi of carbohydrate-aromatic packing interactions in proteins. Journal of the American Chemical Society, 2013, 136: 9877-9866.

[806] Kumar S, Pandya P, Pandav K Gupta SP and Chopra A. Structural studies on ligand-DNA systems: A robust approach in drug design. J. Biosci. 2012, 37: 553-561.

[807] Zhong HA, Arbiser J and Bowen JP. Selectivity, binding affinity and ionization state of matrix metalloproteinase inhibitors. Current Pharmaceutical Design. 2013, 19: 4701-4713.

[808] Beteringhe A, Racuciu C, Balan C, Stoican E and Patron L. Molecular docking studies involving transitional metal complexes (Zn(II), Co(I), Cu(II), Fe(II), Ni(II) with cholic acid (AC) as ligand against Aurora: A Kinase. Advanced Material Research. 2013, 787:236-240.

[809] Pedersen JT and Heegaard. Analysis of protein aggregation in neurodegenerative disease. Analytical Chemistry. 2013, 85: 4215-4227.

[810] Clark JI. Self-assembly of protein aggregates in ageing disorders: the lens and cataract model. Phil. Trans. R. Soc. B 2014, 368:1-7.

[811] Rangappa SK, Quintanova C, Marques SM, Esteves AR, Cardoso SM AND Santos MA. Design and synthesis of tacrine-benzothiazole hybrids as multitarget drugs for Alzheimer's disease, Bioorganic and Medicinal Chemistry 2013, 21: 4558-4669.

[812] Cross JB, Thompson DC, Rai BK, Baber JC, Fan KY, Hu Y,and Humblet C. Comparison of several molecular docking programs: pose prediction and virtual screening accuracy. J. Chem. Inf. Model. 2009, 49: 1455-1474.

[813] Li X, Li Y, Cheng T, Liu Z and Wang R. Evaluation of the Performance of Four Molecular Docking Programs on a Diverse Set of Protein-Ligand complexes. Comput Chem 2010,31: 2109-2125.

[814] Mukherjee S, Ballus TE, Rizzo RC. Docking validation resources: protein family and ligand flexibility ligand flexibility experiments. J. Chem. Inf. Model.2010, 50:1986-2000.

[815] Yuriev E, Agostino M, Ramsland PA. Challenges and advances in computational docking: 2009 in review. J. Mol. Recognit. 2011, 24: 149-164.

[816] Plewczynski D, Lazniewski M, Augustniak R and Ginalski K. Can we trust docking results? Evaluation of seven commonly used programs on PDBbind database. J. Comput. Chem. 2011, 32, 742-1755.

[817] Ripphausen P, Nisius B, Peltason L, Bajorath J. Quo vadis virtual screening? A comprehensive survey of prospective applications. 2010, J. Med. Chem. 53, 8461-8467.

[818] Wallach I, Jaitly N, Nguyen K, Schapira M and Lilien R. Normalizing molecular docking rankings using virtually generated decoys. J. Chem. Inf. Model, 2011, 51: 1870-1830.

[819] Dunbar JB, Smith Richard D, Damm-Ganamet KL, Ahmed A, Esposito E. Xavier DJ, Chinnaswamy K, *et al*, CSAR data set release 2012: ligands, affinities, complexes and docking decoys, J. Chem. Inf. and Mod. 2013, 53: 1842-1852.

[820] Mysinger M, Stoichet BK. Rapid context dependent ligand desolvation in molecular docking. J. Chem. Inf. Model. 2010, 50: 1561-1573.

[821] Malde AK, Mark AE. Challenges in the determination of the binding modes of non-standard ligands in X-ray crystal complexes. J. Comput. Aided Mol. Des. 2011, 25:1-12.

CHAPTER 2

Estimating Protein-Ligand Binding Affinity by NMR

Susimaire Pedersoli Mantoani, Peterson de Andrade, Carlos Henrique Tomich de Paula da Silva

School of Pharmaceutical Sciences of Ribeirão Preto, University of São Paulo, Av. do Café, s/n, Monte Alegre, 14040-903, Ribeirão Preto, São Paulo, Brazil

Abstract: Deep knowledge of how the binding processes occur, such as drug-receptor, signal transduction and cellular recognition, is indispensable for a greater understanding of biological functions. Medicinal chemistry in the path of drug discovery has focused on studies of the molecular interactions which are involved in the development of severe disease state. Thereby, an accurate knowledge about the underlying protein receptor-ligand recognition events at atomic level is fundamental in the process to comprehension, identification and optimization of more potent drug candidates. In this sense, several novel NMR spectroscopic techniques can yield insight into protein-protein interactions in solutions at the molecular level. Resonance signal of the protein or the ligand can be used to identify binding events from a broad range of experiments. For this purpose, changes in NMR spectroscopy parameters such as chemical shifts, relaxation times, diffusion constants, NOEs or exchange of saturation can serve as a measure of binding. In this chapter, the main NMR experimental approaches applied to characterize protein-ligand binding affinity will be discussed. Thus, we hope to provide the reader with a broader and better understanding of how NMR spectroscopy techniques can be applied to a drug discovery process.

Keywords: ^{13}C-labeled protein, ^{15}N-labeled protein, binding affinity, diffusion constant, diffusion ordered spectroscopy (dosy), drug discovery, hsqc (heteronuclear single quantum coherence), intermolecular interaction, nmr screening methods, nuclear magnetic resonance (nmr), nuclear overhauser effects (noe), protein-ligand interaction, relaxation time, std (saturation transfer difference), trosy (transverse relaxation optimized spectroscopy), waterlogsy (water-ligand observed *via* Gradient Spectroscopy).

*Corresponding author Susimaire Pedersoli Mantoani:** School of Pharmaceutical Sciences of Ribeirão Preto, University of São Paulo, Av. do Café, s/n, Monte Alegre, 14040-903, Ribeirão Preto, São Paulo, Brazil; Tel: 55-26-3602-4250; E-mail: smp@usp.br

INTRODUCTION

It is known that most biological processes are essentially dependent on the interactions that occur between macromolecules in the living organisms and small molecules, which can be synthesized or natural compounds. It means that biological functions are promoted or inhibited by the interaction of biomolecules with their ligands. Thus, a deep knowledge of how the binding processes occur (cellular recognition, cell-antigens recognition, hormone-receptor interaction, drug-receptor interaction, *etc.*) is indispensable for a better understanding of the biological systems and even for specific interventions [1-3].

Considering this context, X-ray crystallography and Nuclear Magnetic Resonance (NMR) spectroscopy have been important tools to provide detailed structural information regarding the ligand-target complex. Commonly, X-ray crystallography is used to determine the structure of biological macromolecules, mainly protein and nucleic acids (DNA and RNA), but it is useful only for those that can be coaxed into a crystalline state. However, when a complex cannot be crystallized, NMR spectroscopy can be used to obtain structural information in solution, as it really is in biological systems [1, 4, 5].

Over past decades, NMR spectroscopy ceased to be an analytical technique designed only to investigate the structure of small compounds. In recent years, great improvements in NMR technology have enabled it to be an attractive tool for the study of high- and low-affinity biomolecular interactions between protein-protein, protein-nucleic acid and protein-ligand [6-8]. NMR is considered a versatile biophysical technique since it detects and quantifies molecular interactions in solution at atomic level through experiments that can indicate and characterize binding events by looking at the resonance signals of the ligand or the protein. Besides providing detailed structural information, NMR is unique in its ability to provide thermodynamic and kinetic aspects of a binding reaction in macromolecular complexes [3, 7, 9-11].

Probably, the most impacting and benefiting result of these advances in the NMR spectroscopy has been observed in its wide application in drug discovery process in the academy and pharmaceutical industry. Undoubtedly, the process to identify and optimize drug candidates is long, complex, costly and highly risky once it encompasses several stages (Fig. **1**) [3, 8, 10, 12].

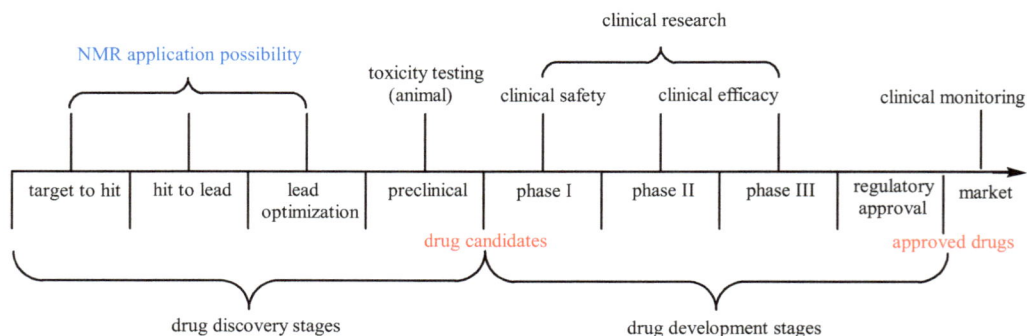

Figure 1: Application of NMR in a general drug discovery process. Figure adapted from (Refs. [9, 13, 14]).

Biomolecular NMR (NMR technology focused on biomolecular interactions) has been implemented in order to provide critical information during early stages in the research of new drugs. The variety of measurable NMR parameters is synergistic with other approaches (combinatorial and medicinal chemistry, high throughput screening (HTS), *in silico* screening, structure-based drug design, *etc*) and allows its application on target identification, hit identification/validation and lead optimization through monitoring protein-ligand interactions [8, 10, 13, 15].

The interactions can be detected by observation of either macromolecule NMR parameters or small molecule NMR parameters. In theory, all NMR spectroscopic parameters may reveal the binding activity between ligands to proteins. For this purpose, parameters such as chemical shift changes, changes in relaxation time, changes of diffusion constant, changes of NOEs (Nuclear Overhauser Effects) or exchange of saturation serve as measures of binding. Nevertheless, only parameters easily obtained and highly sensitivity are relevant. In practice, the determination of structure of a complex by NMR in solution is usually limited by physical properties (solubility and size) and availability ($^{13}C/^{15}N/^{2}D$ labeling from expression systems) regarding the target [3, 5, 16].

In this chapter the main NMR experimental approaches applied to identify and characterize protein-ligand binding affinity will be discussed in order to provide a broader and better understanding of how NMR spectroscopy techniques can be applied to a drug discovery process.

Protein-ligand Binding Affinity and NMR Parameters

First of all, it is important to bear in mind that the affinity of drug for protein is a measure of how strongly that drug binds to the protein [17]. Then, binding affinity can be determined from measurements of dissociation constants (K_D). In a system of the binding of small molecule ligands and large receptor proteins there is a dynamic equilibrium involved, where three species are present: the free receptor (R), the free ligand (L), and the receptor-ligand complex (RL), as represented in Equation 1:

$$[R] + [L] \rightleftharpoons [RL] \tag{1}$$

This equilibrium has an association rate constant (k_{on}) and a dissociation rate constant (k_{off}) (Scheme 1) [7, 14, 18].

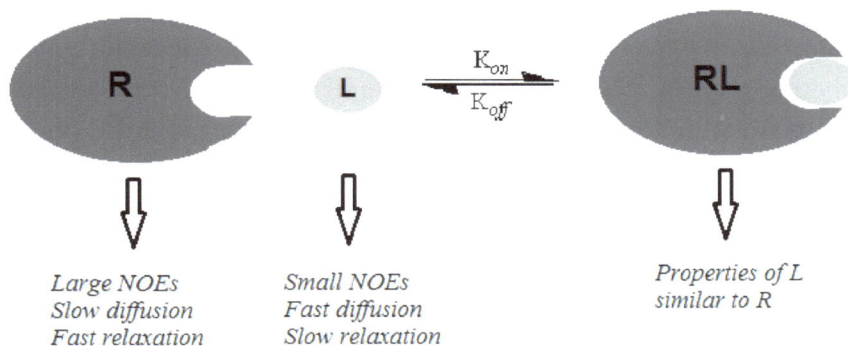

Large NOEs	Small NOEs	Properties of L
Slow diffusion	Fast diffusion	similar to R
Fast relaxation	Slow relaxation	

Scheme 1: NMR properties of receptor (R), ligands (L) and receptor-ligand complex (RL). Scheme adapted from (Refs. [7, 14, 18]).

From this, the binding affinity can be quantified by the temperature-dependent equilibrium dissociation constant (K_D), given by Equation 2 [17]:

$$K_D = \frac{[R][L]}{[RL]} = \frac{k_{off}}{k_{on}} \tag{2}$$

Consequently, the most widely preferred quantitative measure of receptor-ligand binding affinity is dissociation constant K_D, since it is a measurement of stability for bimolecular complexes and its meaning is clear. Moreover, K_D has the units of concentration. Therefore, a value of K_D in mM range indicates a nearly 1:1000 ratio of free to bound states in an equimolar mixture of P and L and a K_D in μM range implies an approximately 1:1000,000 ratio of these states, *i.e.*, the higher the binding affinity, the lower the value of K_D [2].

To determine K_D through NMR experiments it is necessary to perform a quantitative analysis of solutions that are potentially μM in the observed nucleus. When in the free state, the receptor and ligand maintain their individual NMR parameters (*e.g.* chemical shifts, relaxation rates, translational diffusion coefficients). However, when in the bound state, the related binding affinity of ligand and receptor leads to an exchange process that alternates two sets of molecules between the free and bound states.

At equilibrium, the system presents free and bound state populations ([R], [L], [RL]) consistent with Equation 1. In bound state, the ligand transiently adopts NMR parameters characteristic of the typically much larger receptor. On the other hand, analyzing receptor NMR parameters, the ligand briefly perturbs the binding site environment, which may alter distribution of conformations of some receptor molecules group [18]. In both cases, the NMR parameters are influenced by intermolecular interaction. Thus, through NMR experiments may be possible to observe the ligand, the receptor or both, but commonly only one species is chosen as the target of observation. Analyzing the ligand signal it is possible to distinguish between free [L] and bound [RL] ligand, so [L] and [RL] can be quantified. Similarly, observing the receptor it becomes possible to separate quantitatively free [R] and bound [RL] receptor signal [2].

In either case, the interaction modulates the NMR parameters of both molecules. For a system in slow exchange (usually this means a system with high binding affinity and low dissociation constant, K_D = μM or lower), on the chemical shift time scale, distinct signs for the free and bound states, *i.e.*, [L] and [RL] might be observed. However, in practice this is unviable due to the difficulty of detecting signal in μM concentration. Furthermore, in fast exchange systems (system with low binding affinity and high dissociation constant, $K_D > \mu M$) the observed NMR response of the ligand nuclei and the protein is an average between the bound and free states [4].

$$M_{obs} = X_{L(Free)} M_{L\,(Free)} + X_{L(Bound)} M_{L(Bound)} \tag{3}$$

According to Equation 3, M_{obs} is any NMR observable parameter of the equilibrium system, $X_L(free)$ and X_L (bound) are the mole fractions of free and bound ligand, and $M_L(free)$ and M_L (bound) are the NMR parameters of the ligand in its free and bound states, respectively. Likewise for observation of the receptor, where X_R and M_R are now the mole fraction and the NMR parameters of the non-bound and occupied receptor. The mole fractions are defined by Equation 4 [2].

$$M_{obs} = X_{R(Free)} M_{R\,(Free)} + X_{R(Bound)} M_{R(Bound)} \tag{4}$$

When the exchange is very slow on the "NMR timescale" - here relative to the magnitude of the chemical shift difference between the two states - two separate resonances can be seen at the positions corresponding to the chemical shifts characteristic of the two states. At the other extreme, when the exchange is very fast relative to the chemical shift difference, a single resonance will be observed, whose position is the average of the chemical shifts of the two states, weighted by their relative populations (Equation 3). Between these extremes there are complex changes in line shape, which are very sensitive to the precise value of the rate exchange [4].

NMR-Based Methods in Protein-Ligand Binding Affinity

NMR spectroscopy is highly used as a powerful technique to view full details of molecular structures, but in drug discovery its greatest potential is its ability to provide information about intermolecular interactions at the atomic level. This methodology is known as NMR screening. Once a simple parameter, such as the NMR chemical shift, is highly sensitive to environment of the atom, allowing to obtain information about how a small molecule is bound to a macromolecular target, and what parts of the small molecule or which fragments are responsible by interaction [10].

Stockman and Dalvit defined NMR screening as the identification of small molecules ligands for macromolecular targets by observation of a change in an

NMR parameter that occurs upon their interaction [15]. The more common NMR screening techniques used to identify protein-ligand binding affinity are focused on the observation of either protein NMR parameters or ligand NMR parameters. The choice of which path could be used depends on certain conditions, such as the macromolecular target size, availability of protein by recombinant techniques and the K_D complex [1].

At first, all NMR spectroscopy parameters might be able to determine protein-ligand binding; however in practice only parameters easily obtained and highly sensitivity are applied [3]. When protein-based NMR methods are used, the parameter that can be observed is chemical shift changes, after and before interaction with ligand. The greatest advantage of this methodology is that it does not rely on fast exchange to get bound state information, allowing the characterization of both higher and lower binding affinities. Furthermore, by identifying perturbations of assigned chemical shift of protein it is possible to localize and characterize the binding sites [19].

However, the major limitation of this method is the need of milligram quantities of ^{15}N- or ^{13}C-labeled protein soluble and also heteronuclear two-dimensional NMR correlations well-resolved [1]. Thus, in some cases, the time required for NMR assignment of such targets is so large that other techniques, as X-ray crystallography, are favored because they are capable of promoting high-resolution structural information to medicinal chemistry on a faster time scale [19]. Details of protein-based NMR methods will be further discussed.

Another possibility to determine protein-ligand binding affinity is a ligand-based NMR method, which compares parameters of small molecules in the presence and absence of the receptor. In this case, the NMR parameters used are more diversified, including changes in transverse and longitudinal relaxation rates, changes of diffusion constant, changes of NOEs, or exchange of saturation. In turn, for this methodology it is unnecessary to utilize isotopically enriched protein that allows to evaluate different targets more rapidly. Additionally, analysis of signal from ligand NMR spectra is more simplified compared to protein NMR spectra.

Consequently, a disadvantage of ligand-based NMR methods is the incapacity to localize the binding site into the receptor. Moreover, it relies on fast exchanges system which transfers bound state information to the free state, *i.e.* weakly binding ligands are observed, whereas ligands with high affinity will be missed. This requirement leads to the use of large ligand molar excesses, and the consequent risk is that, under these conditions, ligand may start to occupy weaker affinity nonspecific binding sites. Recent advantages and more details in ligand-based methods are discussed below.

Protein-Based NMR Methods

Protein-based NMR methods are based on the chemical shift difference in the resonance signal of the protein atoms when they are interacting or not with the ligand. This methodology relies on the fact that protein chemical shifts are sensitively dependent on both chemical environment of the respective residue and conformational/dynamic changes upon ligand binding [18]. Considering the difficulty to analyse 1D protein spectra due to signal overlapping, HSQC (heteronuclear single quantum coherence) and TROSY (transverse relaxation optimized spectroscopy) [20] experiments are frequently the most used. However, ^{15}N-labeled protein is required to perform these techniques.

All amino acids in ^{15}N-labeled protein, except proline, give rise to single peaks in a ^{1}H-^{15}N HSQC or TROSY spectrum [18]. For ligand binding studies, the NMR spectrum is usually obtained in the absence and presence of a ligand, which is not observed since it is not ^{15}N-labeled. Protein chemical shifts changes indicate binding. Thus, it can be used to identify the location of binding sites in the protein [14].

^{1}H-^{15}N HSQC experiments are limited to smaller proteins (<35 kDa), but the introduction of transverse relaxation optimized spectroscopy (TROSY)-type experiments potentially enables the study of larger protein targets [7].

In some cases, an alternative to ^{15}N, ^{1}H-HSQCs using ^{15}N-labeled protein has been suggested to record ^{13}C-^{1}H correlation spectra with ^{13}C-methyl-labeled protein [21]. On the other hand, to overcome the shortcomings of ^{1}H/^{13}C-HSQC for screening, another technique was suggested to allow only the selective labelling of protons from methyl groups of valin, leucin and isoleucine. This approach significantly reduces the complexity of the resulting HSQC spectra and increases the sensitivity due to the presence of three protons in methyl groups *versus* a single proton in the NH groups. In addition, the favourable relaxation properties of methyl groups also provide the application of this methodology to larger proteins [3]. It is important to note that HSQC-NMR can also contribute to understand the kinetics of complex formation, once the line shapes of peaks in an HSQC spectrum corresponding to the free and bound states are sensitive to on and off rates, especially $k$off [18, 22].

In general, NMR screening methods that monitor the macromolecular target are known as "SAR by NMR" (Structure-Activity Relationship by Nuclear Magnetic Resonance) technique, which is based on the use of chemical shift changes to screen low-affinity ligands, in combination with structural information to direct a linked-fragment approach for achieving binding affinity enhancement [15].

The utility of the SAR by NMR methodology for pharmaceutical research has been demonstrated in a number of systems, including FK506 binding protein (FKBP), metalloproteinase stromelysin [23], and DNA-binding E2 protein from papilloma virus. In the first two cases, compounds with nanomolar affinity were developed by covalently linking fragment molecules with micromolar affinities. The fragment molecules were identified as leads using the SAR by NMR method. The tethering of these two compounds was based on the NMR determined binding sites and known structural information from protein. As an example, a 15 nM inhibitor of stromelysin was discovered by the covalent joining of two weak binders, acetohydoxamic acid (K_D = 17 mM) and 3-(cyanomethyl)-40-hydroxybiphenyl (K_D = 0.02 mM) [24].

Ligand-Based NMR Methods

Ligand-based NMR methods are based on the main difference that exists between protein and ligand, *i.e.* size and volume. Small molecules commonly used as protein inhibitors have molecular masses below 1 kDa, whereas macromolecular proteins have masses usually larger than 10 kDa [25, 26]. These clear differences suggest that it is possible to watch for changes in the ligand NMR relaxation parameters in order to investigate binding.

However, the most important in NMR experiments is that in the exchange between bound and free states, relaxation properties can be transferred to ligands bound to proteins Therefore, relaxation properties of small molecules not binding to proteins differ vastly from those which interact with proteins. While small molecules are characterized by small transverse relaxation rates, weakly positive cross-relaxation rates and large diffusion constants, the opposite can be verified for large molecules. These differences cause line broadening, changes in the diffusion coefficient and an inversion of the nuclear Overhauser effect's (NOE) sign.

From these features, ligand-based NMR experiments were developed to verify the occurrence of intermolecular interactions and identify the region responsible for this interaction with ligand. In general, three main experimental approaches are applied. The first one involves magnetization transfer by NOE, which includes the transferred NOE, NOE pumping and reverse pumping, saturation transfer (STD-NMR), waterLOGSY, among others [28]. The second and third approaches focus on changes in relaxation and diffusion behavior of the ligand upon binding to a protein. In this chapter the most widely used experiments in drug discovery has been reported. In addition, a detailed description of several methods can be found in the literature [1, 2, 7, 15, 19, 25-27].

Approaches Involving Magnetization Transfer

Methods using magnetization transfer are the most popular NMR screening techniques for drug discovery due to several advantages, such as applicability to large protein complexes, need of low protein concentrations and broad applicability.

Magnetization transfer can occur between target and ligand spins in transiently forming complexes through the NOE, which is a manifestation of cross-relaxation between two nuclear spins close to each other in space. The dependence of NOE on the spatial relationship of two nuclei makes it an important tool for studying intermolecular interactions [27]. NOEs connect pairs of hydrogen atoms separated by less than about 5 Å in amino acid residues that may be far away along the protein sequence but close together in space [4].

When small molecules bind to the receptor, the NOEs undergo drastic changes leading to the observation of transferred NOEs (trNOEs). These changes are the basis for a variety of NMR experiments that are designed to detect and characterize an intermolecular interaction [3]. The well-known trNOEs are described by a short correlation time and small positive NOE values for a small molecule (ligand), while a large molecule (receptor) presents a long correlation time and large negative NOE values. Consequently, let us consider a protein-ligand system, where the ligand is present in excess and is in fast chemical exchange. In this case, the large negative NOE acquired by the ligand while it was at the binding site overcomes the small positive NOE of the free ligand (Scheme 2). The observed response will be dependent on the fraction of bound ligand (among some other parameters) [28].

We describe subsequently, some of the NMR techniques based on the trNOE phenomenon that have been used to detect and characterize intermolecular interaction in combinatorial libraries and other complex compound mixtures.

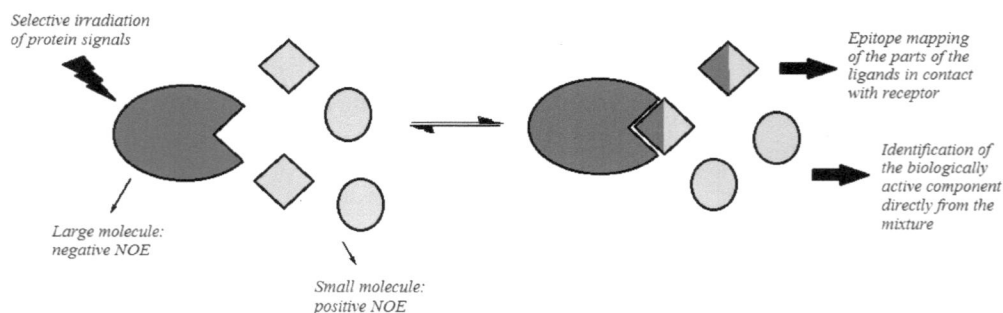

Scheme 2: Schematic illustration of the methods using magnetization transfer. For these experiments, protein resonances are saturated selectively without affecting resonances of the ligand. Compounds that interact (rhombus) with the protein shows the saturation effect (parts of the bound ligand colored in darker gray), which indicate reduced signal intensities. Non-binding molecules (oval circles) are and behave like small molecules. (Adapted from Refs. [3, 26]).

NOE Pumping and Reverse Pumping

In the NOE pumping experiment the magnetization transferred from the receptor to the ligand can be observed, while in its related reverse NOE pumping experiment the reverse process of magnetization transferred from the ligand to the receptor is monitored.

The NOE pumping experiment permits fast and direct detection of ligand binding to target macromolecules without regard for the size of the macromolecule [24]. This method relies on NOE transference magnetization from the protein to the ligand by applying a diffusion filter, which eliminates the signals of the ligand. Consequently, ligand molecules in fast exchange which experience magnetization transfer from the protein can be detected. For example, NOE pumping has been used to detect salicylic acid binding to human serum albumin (HSA) in the presence of non-binding compounds [29].

In the reverse NOE pumping experiment (RNP) a transverse relaxation filter is first applied to attenuate the receptor signal while preserving and inverting the ligand signals. During a mixing time, ligand magnetization is partially transferred to the protein through intermolecular cross-relaxation. A reference experiment in which no magnetization transfer takes place is subtracted. In the difference spectrum, only signals of compounds which interact with the protein are observed [24, 30].

The method has been demonstrated with HSA solutions containing the non-binding small molecule glucose and a series of unbranched fatty acid molecules that are known ligands. Only the fatty acids has beene observed in the difference spectrum. The amount of signal pumped increased with fatty acid chain length, indicative of increasing affinity, suggesting that a series of ligands can be ranked by affinity, using this technique [15, 30].

For identification of weak affinity ligands, the NOE pumping experiment is more robust than the standard diffusion experiments. NOE pumping and reverse NOE pumping are very sensitive experiments for primary NMR screening and the latter is considered to be more sensitive.

Saturation Transfer Difference (STD-NMR)

Saturation transfer difference (STD) NMR spectroscopy, represents one of the most sensitive and versatile ligand-observed NMR screening methods, which is used to detect ligands with binding affinity typically in the micromolar to milimolar range [31]. The basis of this methodology is that the magnetization transfer can occur between the target and ligand spins in transient forming complexes through the NOE.

In STD experiments, a selective radio frequency pulse is applied in a spectral region where no ligand resonances are expected, but the protein is completely saturated due to its larger line width and spin diffusion. Moreover, a ligand that binds to the protein will also be saturated. The degree of ligand saturation naturally relies on the residence time of the ligand in the receptor binding site. Thus, after dissociation, the ligand can be observed in the free state by a reduction of signal intensity compared to a reference spectrum with irradiation far away from any resonance. Therefore, subtracting a spectrum, in which the receptor is saturated, from one without protein saturation produces a difference spectrum in which only the signals of the ligand(s) remain [3, 27, 32].

On the other hand, STD experiments are strongly K_D dependent. In other words, if binding is very tight, the saturation transfer to the ligand molecules is not very efficient. This is common for K_D values lower than 1 nm. On the other hand, if the K_D values are 100 nM or higher, fast exchange of free and bound ligands leads to a very efficient buildup of saturation of the ligand molecules in solution. It is clear that the observed intensity of the signals arising from the ligand in the STD NMR spectrum is not proportional to the binding strength. STD NMR effects depend largely on the off rate, since larger off rates should result in larger STD signals. However, when binding becomes very weak, the probability of the ligand being in the receptor site becomes very low. This results in weak STD signals. STD NMR spectroscopy can be used from very tight binding up to a K_D of about 10 mM [3].

Moreover, the intensity of the STD signals is also dependent on several parameters that can be optimized, such as the receptor concentration, the ligand-receptor concentration ratio and the saturation time [1]. In some cases, the need of a large ligand excess allows STD measurements with very low protein concentrations. A discussion about theses parameters, as well as STD amplification factor, has been reported by Mayer & Meyer [33-36].

One of the advantages of the STD method is that it can be incorporated into two-dimensional experiments, such as two-dimensional STD-TOCSY or STD-HSQC

[3, 36, 37]. In STD experiments, the degree of saturation of ligand resonances depends on the distance of the protons involved, which are saturated to a higher degree when in close proximity to the receptor molecule, thus leading to a stronger STD signal. This information can be used to perform a mapping of the binding epitope (group epitope mapping) [35]. This is important for the directed developments of drugs [4]. Actually, there are several papers in the literature describing STD-NMR as a tool in order to identify the binding epitope, obtain the binding constants, characterize ligand binding to viruses, membrane-integrated proteins and immobilized proteins [3].

WaterLOGSY

The WaterLOGSY (Water-Ligand Observed *via* Gradient SpectroscopY) experiment is a variation of magnetization transfer between protein and ligand, employing the large bulk water magnetization to transfer magnetization *via* the protein-ligand complex to the free ligand, in a selective manner. Magnetization is transferred from water to the protein and to the ligand. It can also be transferred directly from bulk water to the ligand without the pathways through the protein. Meantime, signals of non-binding ligands have opposite sign compared to signals of ligands that bind with high affinity, allowing fast distinction between bound and not bound molecules to the protein [15, 26].

The method is more efficient for ligands displaying dissociation constants in the μM to mM range. Normally, an excess of ligand (10 to 20 fold) with respect to the protein concentration must be used. In addition, it can also be incorporated into two-dimensional NMR experiments. In some cases, optimization of parameters can be obtained by raising the temperature, adding small amounts of organic solvent or by changing the ionic strength [4].

WaterLOGSY experiments have a great potential in primary NMR screening, since the experiment is very sensitive and requires only very low protein and modest ligand concentrations. One disadvantage of this method is that binding and non-binding compounds give signals of opposite phase, resulting in complications concerning crowded spectra, which is very common to combinatorial libraries [11, 26].

Approaches involving Relaxation Time

In NMR spectroscopy the term relaxation is used to describe the process which restores equilibrium magnetization and random phase [26]. There are two distinct relaxation mechanisms, *i.e.* transverse (T2) and longitudinal (T1) relaxation with the respective relaxation rates $R2$ and $R1$. Longitudinal relaxation (T1) is non-selective and can be very similar for small and large molecules whereas transverse relaxation (T2) is quite different [39]. Small ligands tumble rapidly in solution and have small transverse relaxation rates. Large molecules tumble slowly and relax fast. Hence a ligand, bound to a protein, relaxes faster than the unbound ligand [4].

NMR relaxation can be associated with fluctuating electrical fields, originated from the overall tumbling and internal motions of the molecule. The transverse relaxation rate of a nucleus in a molecule is, to a first approximation, proportional to its tumbling correlation time (τc). Since large molecules tumble slowly in solution, the τc of their rotational motion is relatively long, causing large relaxation rates $R2$ and therefore large line widths of NMR signals. Compounds interacting with large molecular weight receptor show broadened lines and increased $R2$ values. Thus, in order to detect binders, compounds line-shapes can be compared in the presence and absence of the receptor, since binding-induced R2 enhancements may be visible by simple line-broadening of proton resonance lines upon addition of the receptor [4, 25, 39].

Another experimental method involving T2 relies on the separate acquisition of spectra from the mixture of compounds in the presence and absence of the protein. Subsequent subtraction leads to spectra containing contribution only from binding ligands [3]. The potential of these methods for NMR screening has been described by Fesik and coworkers. They identified a ligand for FKBP [40] with an affinity of 200 μM from a mixture containing other eight compounds known as FKBP non-binder [41]. On the other hand, T2-filter can be applied to selectively remove signals of the bound ligands to proteins in a mixture of compounds [3, 39]. The increase in relaxation rate can be enhanced tenfold or more by employing spin label coupled to the protein, allowing a reduction in protein concentration [4, 42].

Approaches involving Diffusion Constant

Diffusion NMR related binding studies have two main lines of application, One application is more qualitative, related to the screening of complex mixtures or individual molecules, commonly with the purpose of identifying potential new drug compounds, and another, more quantitative, regarding the determination of association constants [35].

Diffusion is the random translational motion of molecules or ions driven by their internal kinetic energy [35, 43, 44] and it is related to molecular size, as becomes apparent from the Stokes-Einstein equation (Eq. 5)

$$D = k_B T / f \tag{5}$$

where D is the diffusion coefficient, k_B is the Boltzmann constant, T is the temperature, and f is the friction coefficient. For spherical entities the friction factor f is given by

$$f = 6\pi\eta r_H \tag{6}$$

in which η is the viscosity of the solution and r_H is the hydrodynamic (or Stokes) radius of the particle. The Stokes-Einstein equation relates the translational diffusion coefficient at infinite dilution of a spherical particle to its hydrodynamic radius. Thus, from simple equations it is possible to relate experimental diffusion coefficients to molecular radii, Simplicity is the basis for extensive usage [27].

Pulsed field gradient NMR spectroscopy (PFG-NMR) can be used to measure translational diffusion of molecules and also offer an alternative ligand-based approach for studying ligand-protein binding, It can be used for both qualitative and quantitative analysis [27, 35, 45]. The concept of this methodology is very simple and is based on the fact that the diffusion coefficient of a molecule is changed upon addition of another molecule when there is interaction between them [27, 35]. Thus, when a small molecule binds to a large receptor, its diffusion coefficient decreases according to the macromolecule magnitude. It means that the small molecule will have the diffusion coefficient of the large receptor, at least for some time, and if we consider the fast exchange limit, its observed diffusion coefficient (D_{obs}) is described by

$$D_{obs} = x_{free}.D_{free} + x_{bound}.D_{bound}, \tag{7}$$

where xi is the mole fraction.

Thus, when the difference in size between receptor and ligand is large enough, it can be assumed that the diffusion coefficient of the receptor is not largely modified in the free or bound state. However, the diffusion coefficient of the ligand decreases substantially in the bound state, allowing the separation of resonance signals of the complexed molecules from the mixture of the other faster diffusing free ligands [27, 35].

The diffusion ordered spectroscopy (DOSY) NMR technique was introduced by C.S. Johnson Jr. and co-workers [46-48] and has been directly applied to determine the affinity of ligands without the need of titration with ligands. In addition, DOSY can be further combined with other NMR techniques that allows the structural identification of the interacting molecules [45, 49]. Moreover, DOSY-NMR is a powerful tool for analysis of mixtures and identification of receptor binding ligands from a pool of low molecular weight compounds [24]. This technique allows the NMR signals of discrete compounds to be resolved based on variance of translational molecular diffusion rates as well as chemical shifts. Resonances arising from individual chemical species align exactly along the diffusion dimension making it possible to solve mixture components whose diffusion coefficients differ only by a few percent. This makes it of great interest as a tool for analyzing mixtures.

However, NMR diffusion has been used as a tool for spectroscopically isolating and identifying ligands with receptor binding affinity from a mixture of potential ligands. The concept of separating compounds by receptor affinity used in the PFG experiment is reminiscent of affinity chromatography methods and has been termed "Affinity NMR" [24]. The broad applicability of PFG-NMR diffusion measurements is useful since its simplicity makes it flexible to modification. Accuracy in diffusion measurements is improved with modified pulse sequences that permit selective editing or subtraction of undesirable signals, such as the protein background [45].

Modified diffusion experiments can provide a variety of chemical, physical, and structural information. Since PFG-NMR has become a well-established technique for measuring diffusion coefficients and changes in diffusion coefficients for free *versus* bound ligands it is an easy way to probe ligand-protein interactions at the molecular level [45]. However, very weakly bound molecules to the receptor are difficult to be detected since the fraction of bound ligand in the NMR screening experiment will be very small. This removes considerably the expected difference in the diffusion coefficients [3, 35].

CONCLUSION

We have provided the reader with a broader and general understanding of the main NMR experimental approaches applied to identify and characterize protein-ligand binding affinity. NMR techniques for screening have been reviewed in order to present specific aspects regardint their usage in the context of drug discovery and design process [3, 4, 7, 10, 15, 19].

Table 1: Summary of NMR spectroscopy techniques for the identification and characterization of binding of ligands to protein

	SAR by NMR	*NOE pumping*	*STD NMR*	*WaterLOGSY*	*NMR relaxation*	*Diffusion NMR*
Protein (>30kDa)	limited	yes	Yes	yes	yes	no
Protein (<10kDa)	yes	no	No	no	yes	yes
Isotope-labeled protein required	yes	no	No	no	no	no
Binding epitope on protein	yes	no	No	no	no	no
Binding epitope on ligand	no	yes	Yes	yes	no	no
Amount of protein [nmol] at 500 MHz	25	~25	0.1	~25	~1	~100
Identification of ligand	no	yes	Yes	yes	yes	yes

It is important to highlight that both ligand- and receptor-based approaches present advantages and disadvantages. When receptor-based methods are possible, *e.g.* low molecular mass, capable *E. coli* expression *etc*, the potentially higher information content available makes them the right choice. In contrast, ligand-based screening finds broader applicability and places less demands on other research disciplines and infrastructure when there is lack of low-molecular weight drug targets [18]. In Table **1** is a brief summary of the principal NMR techniques discussed in this chapter [3].

ACKNOWLEDGEMENTS

We acknowledge support from CNPq, Fapesp and Capes (Brazil).

CONFLICT OF INTEREST

The authors confirm that this chapter contents have no conflict of interest.

REFERENCES

[1]   Carlomagno T. Ligand-target interactions: what can we learn from NMR? Annu. Rev. Biophys. Biomol.Struct.2005; 34: 245-66.
[2]   Lee Fielding, NMR methods for the determination of protein-ligand dissociation constant. Prog.Nucl.Mag. Res. Sp. 2007; 51: 219-242.
[3]   Meyer B, Peters T. NMR spectroscopy techniques for screening and identifying ligand binding to protein receptors. Angew.Chem. Int. Ed. 2003; 42: 864-890.
[4]   Zerbe O, Mannhold R, Kubinvi H, Folkers G. BioNMR in Drug Research. New York: John Wiley & Sons; 2003.
[5]   Orts J, Griesinger C, Carlomagno T. The INPHARMA technique for pharmacophore mapping: A theoretical guide to the method. J. Magn. Reson.2009; 200: 64-73.
[6]   Bonvin AMJJ, Boelens R, Kaptein R. NMR analysis of protein interaction. Curr.Opin. Chem. Biol. 2005; 9:501-508
[7]   Pellecchia M, Sem DS, Wüthrich K. Nat. Rev. Drug Discov. 2002; 1: 211-219.
[8]   Powers R. Advances in Nuclear Magnetic Resonance for Drug Discovery. Expert Opin Drug Discov. 2009; 4(10): 1077-1098.
[9]   Jahnke W. Perspectives of Biomolecular NMR in Drug Discovery: the blessing and curse of versatility. J. Biomol NMR 2007; 39:87-90.
[10]   Pellecchia M, Bertin, I, Cowburn D, Dalvit C, Giralt E, Jahnke W, James TL, Homans SW, Kessler H, Luchinat C, Meyer B, Oschkinat H, Peng J, Schwalbe H, SiegalG. Perspectives on NMR in drug discovery: a technique comes of ageNat. Rev. Drug Discov. 2008; 7:738-745.
[11]   Salvatella X, Giralt E.NMR-based methods and strategies for drug discovery. Chem. Soc. Rev. 2003; 32: 365-372.

[12]   Lombardino JG; Lowe JA. A guide to drug discovery:The role of the medicinal chemist in drug discovery - then and now. Nat. Rev. Drug Discov. 2004; 3: 853-862.

[13]   Paul SM, Mytelka DS, Dunwiddie CT,Persinger CC, Munos BH, Lindborg SR, Schacht AL. How to improve R&D productivity: the pharmaceutical industry's grand challenge. Nat. Rev. Drug Discov. 2010; 9: 203-214.

[14]   Jahnke W, Widmer H. Protein NMR in biomedical research. CMLS, Cell. Mol. Life Sci. 2004;61: 580-599.

[15]   Brian J, Stockman J, Dalvit C. NMR screening techniques in drug discovery and drug design. Prog.Nucl.Mag. Res. Sp. 2002; 41: 187-231.

[16]   Krajewski M, Rothweiler U, D'Silva L, Majumdar S, Klein C, HolakTA. An NMR-Based Antagonist Induced Dissociation Assay for Targeting the Ligand−Protein and Protein−Protein Interactions in Competition Binding Experiments. J. Med. Chem., 2007; 50: 4382-4387.

[17]   Patrick GL, Spencer J. An Introduction to Medicinal Chemistry.Oxford University Press; 2009.

[18].   Clarkson J, Campbell ID. Studies of protein-ligand interactions by NMR. Biochem. Soc. Trans. 2003; 31: 1006-1009

[19]   Lepre CA, Moore JM, Peng JW. Theory and Applications of NMR-Based Screening in Pharmaceutical Research. Chem. Rev. 2004; 104: 3641−3675

[20]   Riek R, Pervushin K, Wüthrich K. TROSY and CRINEPT: NMR with large molecular and supramolecular structures in solution.Trends Biochem.Sci. 2000; 25: 462-468.

[21]   Hajduk PJ, Augeri DJ, Mack J, Mendoza R, Yang J, Betz SF, Fesik SW. NMR-Based screening of proteins containing ^{13}C-labeled methyl groups. J. Am. Chem. Soc. 2000; 122: 7898 - 7904.

[22]   Ladbury, J.E., Hensmann, M., Panayotou, G. and Campbell, I.D. Alternative Modes of TyrosylPhosphopeptide Binding to a Src Family SH2 Domain: Implications for Regulation of Tyrosine Kinase Activity. Biochemistry 1996; 35: 11062-11069

[23]   Hajduk PJ, Sheppard G, Nettesheim DG, Olejiniczak ET, Shukar SB, Meadows RP, Steinman DH, Carrera GM, Marcotte PA, Severin J, Walter K, Smith H, Gubbins E, Simmer R, Holzman TF, Morgan DW, Davidsen SK, Summers JB, Fesik SW, Discovery of Potent Nonpeptide Inhibitors of Stromelysin Using SAR by NMR. J. Am. Chem. Soc. 1997; 119: 5818 - 5827.

[24]   Shapiro MJ, GounaridesJS. NMR methods utilized in combinatorial chemistry research.Prog.Nucl.Mag. Res. Sp. 1999; 35: 153-200.

[25]   Peng JW, Moore J, Abdul-Manan N. NMR experiments for lead generation in drug discovery.Prog.Nucl.Mag. Res. Sp. 2004; 44: 225 - 256.

[26]   Ludwig C, GuentherUL. Ligand based NMR methods for drug Discovery. Front. Biosci.2009; 14: 4565-4574.

[27]   Brand T, Cabrita EJ, Berger S. Intermolecular interaction as investigated by NOE and diffusion studies. Prog.Nucl.Mag. Res. Sp. 2005; 46: 159-196.

[28]   CraikDJ, WilceJ. Protein NMR Techniques. Springer-Verlag New York, LLC 1997; 60:195-232.

[29]   Chen A, ShapiroMJ. NOE Pumping: A Novel NMR Technique for Identification of Compounds with Binding Affinity to Macromolecules. J. Am. Chem. Soc. 1998; 120: 10258-10259.

[30] Chen A, ShapiroMJ. NOE Pumping. 2. A High-Throughput Method To Determine Compounds with Binding Affinity to Macromolecules by NMR. J. Am. Chem. Soc. 2002; 122: 414-415.

[31] Wang Y, Liu D, Wyss DF. Competition STD NMR for the detection of high-affinity ligands and NMR-based screening. Magn.Reson.Chem. 2004; 42: 485-489.

[32] Milagre CDF, Cabeça LF, Martins LG, Marsaioli AJ. STD NMR Spectroscopy: a Case Study of Fosfomycin Binding Interactions in Living Bacterial Cells.J. Braz. Chem. Soc. 2011; 22: 286-291.

[33] Mayer M, Meyer B. Characterization of ligand binding by saturation transfer difference NMR spectroscopy. Angew.Chem. Int. Ed. 1999; 38: 1784-1788.

[34] Klein J, Meinecke R, Mayer M, Meyer B. Detecting binding affinity to immobilized receptor proteins in compound libraries by HR-MAS STD NMR. J. Am. Chem. Soc. 1999; 121: 5336-5337.

[35] Mayer M, Meyer B. Group epitope mapping by saturation transfer difference NMR to identify segments of a ligand in direct contact with a protein receptor. J. Am. Chem. Soc. 2001, 123, 6108-6617.

[36] Mayer M, Meyer B. A Fast and Sensitive to Method*to* Characterize Ligand Binding *by* Saturation Transfer Difference NMR Spectra.Angew. Chem. 1999, 111, 1902 - 1906.

[37] Vogtherr M, Peters T. Application of NMR Based Binding Assays to Identify Key Hydroxy Groups for Intermolecular Recognition. J. Am. Chem. Soc. 2000, 122, 6093 - 6099.

[38] Meinecke R, Meyer B. Determination of the Binding Specificity of an Integral Membrane Protein by Saturation Transfer Difference NMR: RGD Peptide Ligands Binding to Integrin $\alpha_{IIb}\beta_3$.J. Med. Chem. 2001; 44: 3059 - 3065.

[39] Hajduk PJ, Meadows RP, Fesik SW. NMR-based screening in drug discovery. Q. Rev. Biophys. 1999; 32: 211-240.

[40] Shuker SB, Hajduk PJ, Maeadows RP, Fesik SW. Discovering High-Affinity Ligands for Protein: SAR by NMR. Science, 1996; 274: 1531-1534.

[41] Hajduk PJ, Olejniczak ET, Fesik SW. One-Dimensional Relaxation- and Diffusion-Edited NMR Methods for Screening Compounds That Bind to Macromolecules. J. Am. Chem. Soc. 1997; 119: 12257-12261.

[42] Jahnke W, Rüdisser S, Zurini M. Spin Label Enhanced NMR Screening J. Am. Chem. Soc. 2001; 123: 3149-3150.

[43] Price W.S. Pulsed-Field Gradient Nuclear Magnetic Resonance as a Tool for Studying Translational Diffusion: Part 1. Basic Theory.Concepts Magn.Reson.1997; 9: 299-336.

[44] Nicolay K, Braun KPJ, Graaf RA, Dijkhuizen RM, Kruiskamp MJ. Diffusion NMR spectroscopy.NMR Biomed.2001; 14: 94-111.

[45] Lucas LH, Larive CK. Measuring Ligand-Protein Binding Using NMR Diffusion Experiments. Concepts Magn.Reson. A. 2004; 20: 24-41.

[46] Gibbs SJ, Johnson Jr. C S. A PFG NMR experiment for accurate diffusion and flow studies in the presence of eddy currents J. Magn.Reson.1991; 93: 395 - 402.

[47] Johnson Jr. CS. Diffusion ordered nuclear magnetic resonance spectroscopy: principles and applications. Prog.Nucl.Magn.Reson.Spectrosc.1999; 34: 203 - 256, and references therein.

[48] Wu D, Chen A, Johnson Jr. CS. Flow Imaging by Means of 1D Pulsed-Field-Gradient NMR with Application to Electroosmotic Flow. J. Magn. Reson.Ser.A 1995; 115: 123 - 126.

[49]   Lin M, Shapiro MJ. Mixture Analysis in Combinatorial Chemistry.Application of Diffusion-Resolved NMR Spectroscopy. J. Org. Chem. 1996; 61: 7617 - 7619.

CHAPTER 3

ADME/Tox Predictions in Drug Design

Ricardo Pereira Rodrigues[1], Jonathan Resende de Almeida[1], Evandro Pizeta Semighini[2], Flávio Roberto Pinsetta[1], Susimaire Pedersoli Mantoani[1], Vinicius Barreto da Silva[3], Carlos Henrique Tomich de Paula da Silva[1]

[1]School of Pharmaceutical Sciences of Ribeirão Preto, University of São Paulo, Ribeirão Preto, SP, Brazil; [2]Ribeirão Preto Medical School, University of São Paulo, Ribeirão Preto, SP, Brazil and [3]Catholic University of Goiás, Goiânia, Brazil

Abstract: Most drug candidate failures during clinical trials occur due to inappropriate ADMET properties. In this way, there is a major concern to identify possible ADMET failures during the early stages of drug design projects and optimize such properties in order to reduce time and costs. *In silico* ADMET predictions comprise various strategies that play a central role when considering the task of profiling lead compounds regarding potential ADMET failures. We will discuss the computational strategies, methods and softwares used, actually, to profile ADMET and how they could be helpful during drug design.

Keywords: Absorption, ADME properties, bioavailability, distribution, drug design, excretion, hydrogen bond acceptors, hydrogen bond donors, *in silico* predictions, Ionization constant, lipophilicity, LogP, metabolism, rule of five, software, solubility, toxicity.

INTRODUCTION

The constant evolution of organic chemistry has accelerated the process of lead discovery, contributing to the development of new drugs. However, this process is still long and expensive, with growing costs as the process advances through clinical trials [1]. Nevertheless, the majority of promising leads are eliminated due to unfavorable ADME/Tox (Absorption, Distribution, Metabolism, Excretion and Toxicity) properties, which stimulates the evaluation of these properties during

*****Corresponding author Ricardo Pereira Rodrigues:** School of Pharmaceutical Sciences of Ribeirão Preto, University of São Paulo, Ribeirão Preto, SP, Brazil; Tel: 55-16-3602-0664; E-mail: rpr@fcfrp.usp.br

the early stages of drug development, reducing costs and time, driving researchers to compounds with better viability to debut as a drug [1].

The development of a new drug starts with around 10 thousand compounds and 10% (1,000) of these compounds have good ADMET and safety properties for clinical trials. 1% (10) of these 1,000 may be approved in clinical trials, becoming drug candidates, and around 10% of this, 10 drug candidates, get to the market as a drug after regulatory agencies approval. These long years of work do not guarantee their success due to constant withdrawal of drugs from the market resultant from unacceptable side effects (in some cases, death) that are not identified in clinical trials [2].

The ADME/Tox properties enables adjustment of the therapeutic profile of a new compound, especially during its development. The absorption properties can define if the compound will be used orally, by intramuscular injection or by other route. Likewise, the distribution affects the efficiency of this compound, since it must reach the site where it is supposed to act. With an adequate bioavailability, the metabolism, excretion and toxicity properties of a drug help to determine the efficiency, drug administration intervals, interaction with other substances and side effects. All these properties can shape or even stop the development of a new compound as a drug [3].

In silico predictions have become a very attractive approach in order to model and evaluate ADME/Tox properties when compared to traditional experimental methods due to its lower cost and faster data prospection. *In silico* data can be evaluated even before the compound's synthesis or biological assays, avoiding the ethical barriers of biological trials with animals, saving time and money in the evaluations of compounds that would not reach the market [4].

The major disadvantage of current *in silico* methods is the dependence on a solid data set obtained from experimental procedures. Such data is hard to obtain due to the wide complexity and the diversity of biological systems, nullifying substantial data obtained with animal models or *in vitro* assays (equivalent to humans) [1, 3, 5, 6].

Although *in silico* ADME/Tox predictions grow constantly as a viable alternative, their success is still limited to cases where the query compounds are similar to those with already characterized ADME/Tox properties [1, 3, 5, 6]. Despite these drawbacks, *in silico* methods are in constant improvement aided by new ADME/Tox variable studies. They are becoming a useful and viable tool in drug development [7].

This chapter will focus primarily on absorption, metabolism and toxicity predictions, focusing on the computational strategies, methods and commonly used softwares to profile ADMET predictions and how could they be a useful tool in drug design strategies.

ABSORPTION

Absorption is the process in which a drug enters the bloodstream without being chemically altered in order to be available to reach its site of action in sufficient quantity [8]. In order for a drug to perform a therapeutic effect, it has to be taken to the bloodstream passing through various *in vivo* barriers such as the digestive tract (intestinal absorption), and reach specific tissues or organs [9].

The possible routes for a drug entering the body are: a) enteral; b) parenteral and c) topical. The enteral route includes processes in which the drug is administered through the gastrointestinal tract by sublingual (drug placed under the tongue), oral (swallowing the drug) and rectal (drug absorption occurs in the rectum) via. Parenteral routes are administration routes of a drug that do not involve the digest tract. In this route, drugs are administered by intravascular (drug administered directly into the bloodstream), intramuscular (drug injected in skeletal muscle), subcutaneous (drug absorption from subcutaneous tissue) injection and inhalation (absorption through the lungs). Topical administration involves dosing for mucous membranes (eye drops, antiseptic, sunscreen, for nasal passages, *etc.*) and skin by dermal (oil or ointment – local action) and transdermal (drug absorption through the skin – systemic action) route. Formulations of a drug can be developed to increase the absorption of molecules and this is achieved by increasing the solubility or dissolution rates of the drug product [10].

The most convenient way for patients to receive medications is by the oral route. For a drug orally administered, a high and stable bioavailability is crucial for its successful development. When the drug is orally administered it has to be absorbed through the epithelium of the small intestine [11]. In this case, the drug has to cross several membranes and barriers before reaching its primary site of action. In this process some major factors that affect the absorption are involved, such as the chemical degradation and metabolism of the drug in the gastrointestinal tract and the efflux by P-gp transmembrane transporters [8].

The oral absorption computational prediction area has received concentrated efforts since the oral bioavailability is one of the most desirable attributes of a new drug and the first step to achieve oral bioavailability is to get a good oral absorption [12]. This prediction is very challenging due to the fact that the bioavailability is a complex function of many biological and physicochemical factors [13].

The bioavailability (%F) itself is used to describe the degree to which a drug or other substance becomes available to the target tissue after its administration. When a drug is administered intravenously its bioavailability is 100%. However, when a drug is administered by other routes (such as orally), its bioavailability (oral bioavailability) is usually less than 100% due to degradation or metabolism of the drug prior to absorption, incomplete absorption and first-pass metabolism (first-pass clearance or presystemic metabolism). Before the drug reaches the general circulation, first-pass metabolism clears the absorbed drug, thereby becoming one of several other factors that limit bioavailability. A drug only has oral bioavailability if it can reach the systemic circulation not only flowing through the intestine, but also through the liver because drugs that are orally administered must pass through the liver before reaching the general circulation and some of these compounds are strongly metabolized through the liver (first-pass effect) [13].

During the absorption process a fraction of the drug is lost; such loss is closely related to the liver (metabolic, biliary) and intestine wall by liver cells or enzymatic hydrolysis reactions (intestinal metabolism), respectively. Another enzymatic reaction takes place in the plasma by hydrolytic enzymes in the blood (plasma decomposition) for those molecules that survive in the liver. First-pass effect or presystemic metabolism represents the presystemic drug elimination which occurs during the first-pass through the liver where the concentration of a drug is highly reduced. Drugs such as imipramine, morphine, propranolol, diazepam, cimetidine and lidocaine have a reduced bioavailability due to the presystemic metabolism [10, 14].

Hence, it is important to distinguish between oral bioavailability and absorption, whereas the oral bioavailability is the ratio of both the absorption and the hepatic first-pass metabolism. Therefore, the main difference between absorption and bioavailability is the amount of drug eliminated by secretion or first-pass metabolism through the liver [9].

The GIT absorption process can be altered by several factors, classified into three main classes:

- physicochemical (pKa, solubility, chemical stability, diffusivity, lipophilicity and salt form);

- physiological (gastrointestinal pH, gastric passage, small and large intestine transit time, active transport and efflux, and gut wall metabolism);

- formulation factors (drug particle size and crystal form, and dosage form such as a solution, tablet, capsule, suspension, emulsion, gel, and modified release).

Regarding absorption studies the major efforts are focused on the physicochemical properties of compounds, because the physiological factors cannot be controlled and the formulation specificities are usually experimentally optimized. The main mechanism for drug absorption through intestinal epithelium is passive diffusion driven by a concentration gradient. Depending on the molecule's hydrophobicity, passive diffusion can occur through the lipid/aqueous environment of the cell membrane (trans-cellular transport) or the passage through the water-filled tight junctions formed by the fusion of the lipid membranes of adjacent cells (paracellular transport). In addition, molecules that enter the cytoplasm of epithelial cells can be actively transported back by specific transporters to the intestinal lumen; this efflux process is mainly a function of a transporter in the cell membrane called P-glycoprotein (P-gp) [15].

The field of predicting oral absorption was first defined by the Rule of Five proposed by Lipinski *et al.* [16]. The Rule of Five established guidelines for the identification of compounds with possible low absorption and permeability:

1. molecular weight < 500;

2. calculated logP < 5 (CLOGP) or Moriguchi logP < 4.15 (MLOGP);

3. number of hydrogen bond donors (OH and NH groups) < 5;

4. number of hydrogen bond acceptors (N and O atoms) < 10.

A drawback of the Rule of Five is that it can give only a very limited classification of molecules. Nowadays, many models for prediction of human intestinal absorption (HIA) are available, applying a variety of statistical and machine-learning approaches which include multiple linear regression, nonlinear regression, partial least square regression, linear discriminant analysis, classification and regression trees, artificial neural networks (ANNs), genetic algorithms (GAs), support vector machines (SVMs), so on. Considering that physicochemical properties are related to intestinal absorption, many physicochemical descriptors were introduced in the prediction of HIA, such as polar surface area (PSA), partition coefficients, molecular size, hydrogen bonding descriptors, topological descriptors, and even quantum chemical descriptors [13].

Molecular descriptors to predict the intestinal absorption or oral bioavailability are used as variables to generate prediction models. Molecular descriptors can be divided into three main categories, due to their dependence on the dimensionality of the structural representation:

1. 1D descriptors (depend on the formula of the molecule and can only give information on the composition of the element or molecular weight);

2. 2D descriptors (obtained from the connectivity graph or a molecular graph);

3. 3D (include three-dimensional geometric information of a molecule).

Currently, only one 1D descriptor, the molecular weight (MW), is useful during absorption and bioavailability prediction. Regarding 2D descriptors there are several options, as they are quickly calculated. 2D descriptors include topological polar surface area (TPSA), number of hydrogen bond acceptors (NHBA), number of hydrogen bond donors (NHBD), number of hydrogen bond donors and acceptors (NHD), octanol-water partitioning coefficient (logP), apparent partition coefficient (logD), intrinsic solubility (logS), number of rotatable bonds (Nrot), number of molecular fragments, electrotopological state index (E-state), and a variety of other topological parameters. Lastly, the 3D molecular descriptors most widely used include Polar Surface Area (PSA), molecular surface area (MSA) and molecular volume (MV) [9].

Hou *et al.* [4] studied the performance of a support vector machine (SVM) to classify compounds with high or low fractional absorption (%FA > 30% or %FA ≤ 30%). For this, 10 models of SVM classification were considered to investigate the impact of different individual molecular properties on %FA. Among them were the topological polar surface area (TPSA), octanol-water patitioning coefficient (logP), apparent partition coefficient at pH = 6.5 (logD6.5), number of violations of the Rule of Five (Nrule-of-five), number of hydrogen bond donors (NHBD), number of hydrogen bond acceptors (NHBA), intrinsic solubility (logS), number of rotatable bonds (Nrot), molecular volume (MV), and molecular weight (MW). The database used for analysis consisted of 648 chemical compounds of which 579 molecules were believed to be transported by passive diffusion.

First, the 10 classification models were built using each descriptor individually. The RBF kernel function was used in the analysis of SVM. Subsequently, a validation procedure (1000 times training) was applied for each SVM classifier for each 455 molecules randomly divided into a training group (24 HIA- and 203 HIA+) and a validation group (23 HIA- and 204 HIA+). The 10 SVM classifiers were then ranked according to an average of 1000 times training. Among the 10 molecular descriptors studied, TPSA showed the best performance rating. The TPSA was assumed to be related to the ability of hydrogen bonding and, thus, can be considered for the interaction between drug molecules and the intestine. The SVM model using the TPSA was able to correctly identify 93.1% of the compounds HIA+ (chemical agents absorbable; good-absorption) and 81.4% of the compounds HIA- (non-absorbable; poor-absorption) for validated compounds concluding that taking advantage of a high quality database it is possible to develop a reliable model of SVM to discriminate compounds that are well absorbed and compounds that are poorly absorbed. In addition, such procedure indicates that passive diffusion of intestinal absorption can be well predicted by simple molecular descriptors [4].

There is also, beyond the prediction of human intestinal absorption, a great interest in predicting intestinal permeability. In order to obtain a rapid assessment of intestinal permeability, *in vitro* systems such as Caco-2 monolayers are investigated as potential models for drug absorption. The Caco-2 monolayer is the most advanced *in vitro* cell line model serving as a model for both paracellular and transcelular pathways. The ability of Caco-2 cells to differentiate and form tight junctions between cells justifies them as a model for the paracellular movement of compounds through the monolayer. In addition, Caco-2 cells express transporter proteins, efflux proteins and phase II conjugation enzymes to model a variety of transcelular pathways [17].

Nuez *et al.* [15] summarized from literature, software packages that are commercially available to predict the fraction of human intestinal absorption based on estimates of solubility and intestinal permeability (Table **1**).

GastroPlus program from Simulation Plus Inc. is a software package which performs *in silico* predicted drug absorption model. This program is used for building and optimizing absorption attributes to predict the rate, oral and intravenous absorption, often used to as a tool to identify parameters that could potentially enhance the bioavailability of a compound as well. Some mechanisms are implemented in GastroPlus like gastrointestinal simulation technology (GIST), and Advanced Compartmental Absorption Transit (ACAT) model based upon an original CAT model first elucidated by Yu *et al.* [18], this method is based on nine compartments comparable to the different portion of the digestive tract, among them are seven compartments of the small intestine and colon. Kocic and coworkers [19] reported that the GIST model was used to give a close prediction of LT4 oral absorption. Levothryroxine (LT4) is a drug orally administered used as alternate therapy in primary hypothyroidism. The simulated studies were comparable with the data observed in the *in vivo* bioequivalence study, thus demonstrating that the GIST model gives an accurate indicator of LT4 oral absorption.

Table 1: Programs for *in silico* predictions of human intestinal absorption

Software	Purpose and/or function
GastroPlus (Simulation-plus, Inc. http://www.simulation-plus.com)	Simulates gastrointestinal absorption and pharmacokinetics for drugs administered orally or intravenously in human and animals. Makes predictions of the first-passage effect in the gut and liver and plasma concentration-time profiles. As well as simulations and predictions of bioavailability and pharmacodynamics.
iDEA (LionBioscience, Inc. http://www.lion-bioscience.com/)	Simulates human physiology and explains regional variations in intestinal permeability, solubility, surface area and fluid motion. Absorption module predicts the fraction dose absorbed over time, mass absorbed, soluble mass, insoluble mass, absorption rate and intestinal drug concentration.

To model the absorption of a lipophilic BCS (biopharmaceutical classification system) Class II compound metabolized by CYP3A4 which may be administered as a nanosuspension formulation, Gastroplus software program was used to study the absorption attributes of the compound using the Advanced Compartmental Absorption Transit (ACAT) model implemented in Gastroplus. In this case, the program was used for building and optimizing the PBPK (Physiologically Based Modeling) model to predict the rate and oral absorption in rats by modeling the absorption of nanosuspension. The disadvantage of using GastroPlus for this approach was that the absorption of the nanosuspension formulation could not be favorably modeled, but the PBK model in rats gave a good fit as result for both intravenous and oral dosing [20].

IDEA is another software tool from Lions Bioscience Inc. that acting like human physiology and has models for intestinal permeability, solubility, surface area and fluid movement. This approach for absorption module was based on simulations models to predict oral drug absorption described by Grass [21]. According to this work, they discuss that broad models for oral absorption have the potential to provide substantial benefits to the discovery process and as a result, a significant impact on the yield potential. These models allow direct extrapolation to humans from data measured *in vivo*, thus IDEA makes an *in vitro* determination for the estimation of ADME properties [21].

Parrot and Lavé [22] made an assessment of two software tools that apply physiologically based models for prediction of intestinal absorption in human, GastroPlus and IDEA. They were compared to predict oral absorption describing a comparative evaluation and a discussion of the usability and functionality using, for this purpose, a set of 28 drugs. For pure *in silico* prediction, in terms of ability, both programs were around 70% correct classification rate (71% for IDEA and 68% for Gastroplus) into high ($\geq$66%), medium (between 33-66%) and low ($\leq$33%) category of absorption, in other words, there was no significant difference in performance between them. An improvement in predictive accuracy was observed using IDEA for CACO-2 permeability, whereas GastroPlus did not show any enhancement in predicting, independent of the *in silico* or experimental permeability used.

Here the process was highlighted in which all drugs need to pass to be absorbed and some progress *in silico* modeling of absorption and oral bioavailability. A brief summary of the methodological point of view, as well as some advantages and disadvantages of the programs used to predict human intestinal absorption has been presented as well. Some variables can affect bioavailability and consequently drug absorption such as site of drug absorption, membrane transporters and presystemic drug metabolism. Although there are several *in silico* methods that can be useful in predicting absorption properties for drug design, there is not a general methodology for the computer prediction of absorption properties.

COMPUTATIONAL APPROACHES IN METABOLISM

Most of drug discovery projects are faced with stability limitations in developed series of compounds causing new drugs to be dismissed. Many pharmacologically interesting molecules are passed over because they are not stable enough. These issues have contributed to the development of new strategies for structural modifications focusing in improved stability of future promising compounds [10]. In order to accelerate the development of active compounds, metabolic considerations were integrated into drug design and lead-optimization strategies, comprising the evaluation of chemistry and biochemistry metabolic reactions and their role in the activation/deactivation process. The efficiency of these processes can be improved by *in silico* methods in order to provide reliable and versatile metabolic predictions [23].

Cellular metabolism is characterized as an interlaced network of interactions involving several levels of regulation. This system has a very complex behavior and thus cannot be predicted with only an intuitive approach. However, mathematical models of cellular metabolism are able to create an appropriate framework to represent and investigate different stages of metabolism [24-26]. The statistical methods used to search correlations include multiple linear regression analysis, multivariate analysis, and unsupervised machine-learning approaches, neural networks and genetic algorithms. Thus, a computational approach adopts a hierarchy of descriptions involving different levels of detailed and precise information [23, 27].

The most important enzymes involved in human metabolism are the cytochrome P450. Despite the fact that 57 active genes for CYP are known, only a few enzymes with different prevalence in the human liver are directly related to metabolism. The cytochrome P450 enzymes are a superfamily of heme-thiolateproteins responsible for catalyzing the oxidation of many endogenous and foreign substrates in the body. Danielson and coworkers estimated that 75% of all drugs are metabolized by cytochrome P450 enzymes, highlighting the importance of potential metabolism sites prediction. This is highly advantageous if performed early in the new drug development process. *In silico* modeling of metabolism properties can be performed using many different approaches. However, the metabolism properties are difficult to predict due to multiple physiological processes resulting from the intestinal absorption and metabolic stability [28-31].

The early prediction of ADME properties is strategic since it increases the success rate of compounds reaching the pharmaceutical market. In general the programs perform a comparison of methods (based on pattern recognition) to identify possible correlations between molecular descriptors and ADME properties, structural models based on classical molecular mechanics and quantum mechanical techniques for modeling chemical reactions [32].

In addition to cytochrome P450, other drug metabolizing enzymes and carriers play an important role in drug-drug interactions. According to Boulenc and Barberan [33] there is a growing appreciation for the ratio of transport proteins and drug-drug interactions.

There is a diverse number of softwares used to predict metabolism. Among those commonly used are Meteor [23], MetabolExpert [34], MetaSite [5].

Meteor is a software-based rule, many of these empirical. Their algorithm involves three steps. First, the program examines the lead compound and verifies the existence of variable substructures related to any one of biotransformations contained in its database. Second, through pre-established rules, Meteor assesses the chance of biotransformation, based on five levels that are dependent on the molecule's analyzed logP: probable, plausible, equivocal, doubtful and unlikely [35]. Finally, a score of biotransformations that may occur concomitantly in the same compound are performed. The result of this score is based on a set of established rules, for example, chemical properties inherent in each molecule and functional group's specific features [36].

The software MetaSite (Fig. **1**) predicts metabolic transformations related to cytochrome-mediated reactions in phase 1 metabolism, which encompasses modification of the molecular structure itself, such as oxidation or dealkylation.

Based on the GRID descriptors for cytochrome P450 enzymes and substrate potential [5], metabolism can be assessed at all possible sites of the molecular structure by assigning each atom a probability of metabolism [30]. The accuracy of the program exceeds more than 85%, providing the metabolites structure obtained in a ranking derived from the site of metabolism predictions. The method highlights the atoms in the molecule that contribute to the prediction, directing the molecule in the cytochrome cavity. Modifying the contributing regions that influence mostly the site of metabolism can avoid inhibitory issues such as the direct blocking of the primary site of metabolism, which could create a cytochrome inhibitor.

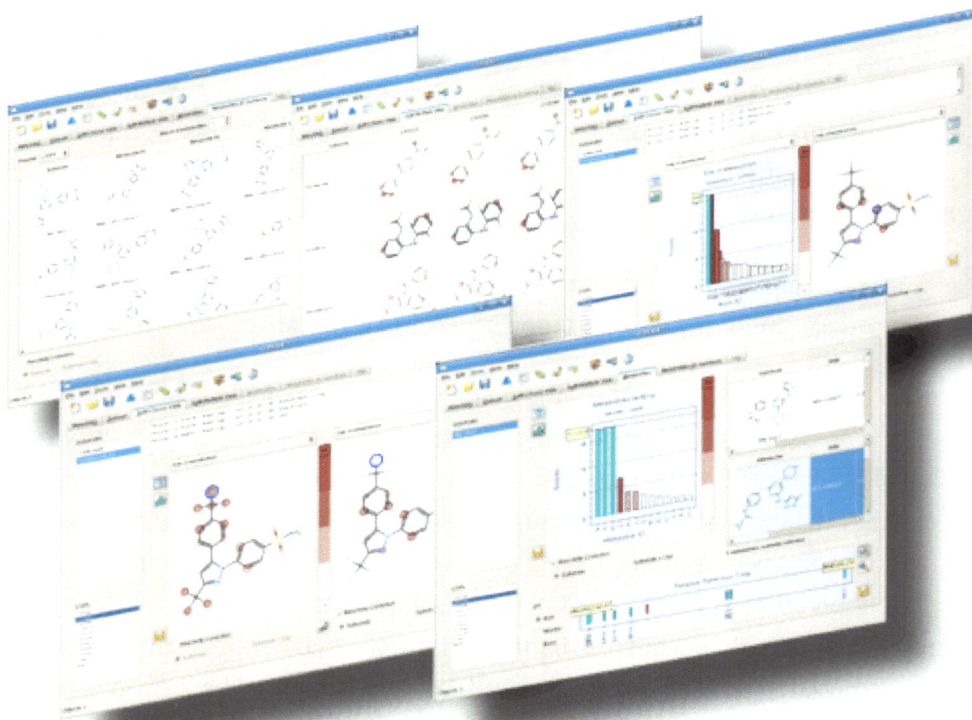

Figure 1: Metasite metabolism prediction (http://www.moldiscovery.com/soft_metasite.php).

As part of an earlier project begun in 1985 by CompuDrug, MetabolExpert was developed with the goal of creating a model for the prediction of chemical transformations in living systems or in a controlled environment, using an expert system approach. This program contains a family of expert systems, each comprising one or more databases, as well as tools for prediction. These databases are composed mostly of metabolic patterns obtained from already created databases and frequent metabolic patterns. Biotransformations were implemented as rules based on the presence or absence of substructures. These rules operate on the original list of molecules (input) to produce first generation metabolites, and the process is repeated until the generation of second generation metabolites [37].

These programs should be used in conjunction with some computer-aided toxicity prediction based on quantitative structure-toxicity relationships or expert systems for toxicity evaluation [38, 39]. Although several studies have been conducted to predict the site of metabolism, there is no consensus on which method is the best. Recent research suggests that the prediction of the metabolism site can be accomplished by estimating the intrinsic reactivity of ligand atoms. This can be estimated using Hartree-Fock methods such as, AM1 or quantum mechanical calculations using DFT approaches [30].

TOXICITY

Toxicity can be defined as any harmful effect of a chemical compound on a target organism [38]. Toxicology is a rather different matter compared with the other ADME disciplines because many different mechanisms may be involved [40]. It is widely accepted that the ionization constant, lipophilicity and solubility are parameters that can affect toxicological aspects [41]. A problem associated with predictions of toxicological effects is that similar compounds may exert their toxicity through different mechanisms [40].

Computational toxicology is an emerging interdisciplinary field that combines *in vitro* assay data with computational approaches to model, understand, and predict the toxicity of environmental chemicals and pharmaceuticals. The need for computational methods is due to the innumerous environmental chemicals without relevant associated toxicity data for estimating potential risks to humans as well as the ethical difficulties and high costs of performing animal-based studies. Moreover, many experimental tests often do not provide the necessary molecular mechanism information required to understand how to extrapolate to human toxicity risk [42].

In silico techniques for the prediction of toxicological endpoints are highly desired in the drug discovery industry because of their fast return of results, inexpensiveness, the advantage of identifying problematic candidates and evaluation metabolites safeness before synthesis [43-46].

Toxicity is responsible for many compounds failing to reach the market and for the withdrawal of a significant number of compounds from the market once they have been approved. In 2003, it was estimated that approximately 20 to 40% of drug failures in investigational drug development could be attributed to toxicity problems. Five years later, toxicity was still the cause of 20% of the dropouts during late development stages [3, 44].

ADME/Tox *in silico* models can fail due to the expectations of the users or due to the development aspects of the model, such as choice of statistical tool, description of the investigated structures and limited model validation [40]. To develop predictive *in vivo* toxicity models based on *in vitro* or *in silico* inputs, large, high-quality collections of animal data are required for training and qualification, and unfortunately much of the world's *in vivo* animal testing data is widely dispersed [42].

There are basically two main *in silico* approaches commercially available to forecast potential toxicity. One approach uses expert systems (ES) that derive models on the basis of abstracting and codifying knowledge from human experts and the scientific literature. The other approach relies primarily on the generation of descriptors of chemical structure and statistical analysis of the relationships between these descriptors and the toxicological end-point, such as carcinogenicity [3, 44]. Benfenati and Gini [38] classified the toxicity preview programs into three categories: Rule-based human-derived ES (DEREK), ES using statistical procedures (TOPKAT and CASE) and ES encoding mechanistic processes (COMPACT).

DEREK (Deductive Estimation of Risk from Existing Knowledge) is the example of an approach based on human expert's knowledge, which evaluates an unknown chemical looking at its similarity with other molecules. It is a qualitative tool used in agrochemical, pharmaceutical and regulatory organizations. DEREK also takes into account physicochemical properties such as log P and pKa. There are several toxicological endpoints including mutagenicity, carcinogenicity, skin sensitization, irritation, reproductive effects, neurotoxicity and others [38, 44, 47-49].

The TOPKAT (Toxicity Prediction by Komputer Assisted Technology) program uses QSAR principles, involving statistical methods such as linear multiple regression equations. It assesses the toxicity of chemicals from their two dimensional (2D) molecular structure. Each module consists of a specific database for predicting a specific toxicity endpoint. The lack of transparency in association of descriptors with toxicity makes TOPKAT marginally useful for consideration of the mechanisms of toxicity [38, 49, 50].

COMPACT (Computer Optimized Molecular Parametric Analysis of Chemical Toxicity) is a structural-based procedure for the prediction of potential toxicity and metabolism *via* P450 enzymes. Compared with the other ES, this is conceptually a different approach, which tends to consider the mechanism of the toxic action. These approaches are related to the known characteristics of biochemical processes, so these systems should greatly improve as knowledge of the biochemical pathways and the structure of the macromolecules involved increases everyday [38, 51].

CASE (Computer Automated Structure Evaluation) is a hybrid of 2D QSAR and artificial expert structure based program. CASE, with its general applicability, has been used for several different classes of chemicals, biological and toxicological activities. The fundamental assumption of its methodology is that if a substructure is relevant to the observed activity, it will be found predominantly in active and marginally active compounds. The program statistically identifies the most significant substructure that exists within the learning set, which consists of inactive and active chemicals. The molecules containing this fragment are then removed from the database, and the remaining molecules are submitted to a new analysis, leading to the identification of the next significant fragment [38, 49, 52].

New free tools in the toxicoinformatics field are available online, based on 2D descriptors, such as LAZAR (http://lazar.in-silico.de/predict), ToxPredict (http://apps.ideaconsult.net:8080/ToxPredict) and CAESAR (http://www.caesar-project.eu/software/index.php). LAZAR (Lazy Structure-Activity Relationships) is an experimental version based on OpenTox, whose linear fragments of the query structure or in one of the training structures are determined exhaustively by molecular feature algorithm (MOLFEA). CAESAR is based on WEKA algorithms [53-55].

WEKA (Waikato Environment for Knowledge Analysis) is a free software available under the GPL (General Public License), developed at the University of Waikato, New Zealand (Fig. **2**). It has a collection of machine learning algorithms for data mining tasks [56]. MOLFEA (Molecular Feature Miner) is a domain specific inductive database which mines for fragments in chemicals. The compounds are stored in the SMILES (Simplified Molecular Input Line Entry System) format and fragments are formulated in the SMARTS language [57].

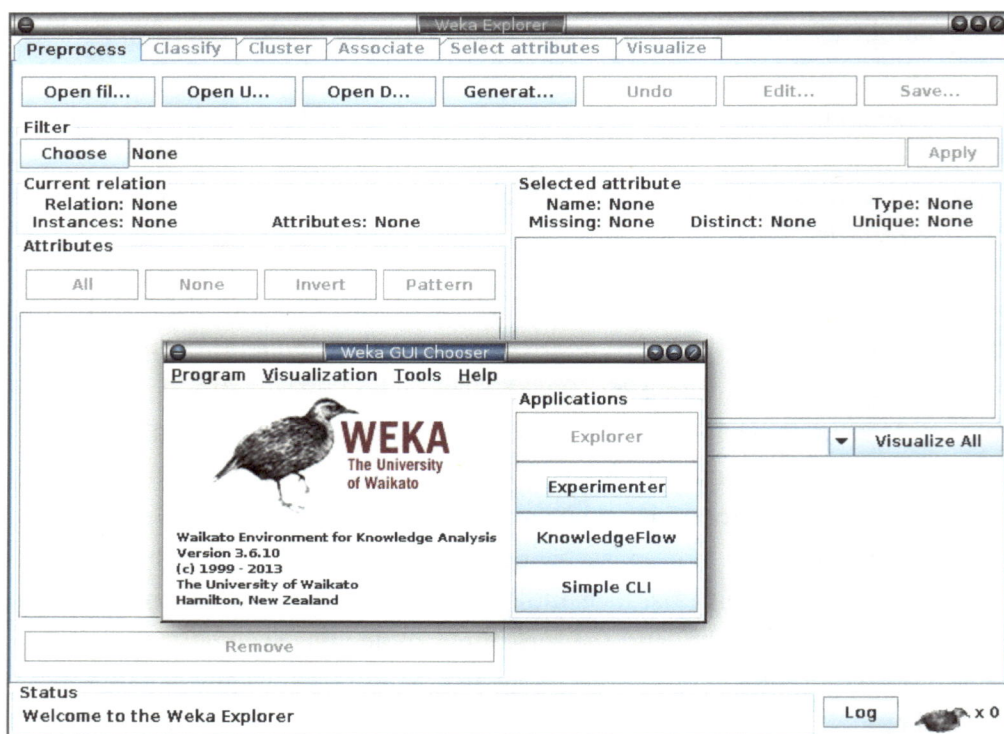

Figure 2: The Weka Software. Weka is a collection of machine learning algorithms for data mining tasks (http://www.cs.waikato.ac.nz/ml/weka/).

Another approach is based on Inverse Docking, a method used for finding proteins associated with potential toxicity and side effect that bind with a specific ligand. INVDOCK uses a flexible docking algorithm to find potential toxicity targets of a small molecule [53]. Another software based on inverse docking is PharmMapper, a freely web server (http://59.78.96.61/pharmmapper/) that provides an *in silico* target prediction method for a given compound by prospecting the potential ligand binding sites stored in potential drug target database, which can be related to toxicity [58].

Therefore, it would be interesting to use more than one activity prediction software, in the search for a new drug, with different methodologies, which makes the results more reliable. This can reduce costs and risks related to drug candidates that are discontinued in advanced clinical phases, due to toxicity problems.

ACKOWLEDGEMENTS

We acknowledge financial support from FAPESP and CNPQ.

CONFLICTS OF INTEREST

The authors confirms that this chapter contents have no conflict of interest.

REFERENCES

[1] Yamashita F, Hashida M, *In Silico* Approaches for Predicting ADME Properties of Drugs, Drug Metabolism and Pharmacokinetics, 2004, 19(5):327-38.

[2] Li AP, *In vitro* approaches to evaluate ADMET drug properties, Current Topics in Medicinal Chemistry, 2004, 4(7):701-6.

[3] van de Waterbeemd H, Gifford E, ADMET *in silico* modelling: towards prediction paradise? Nature Reviews Drug Discovery, 2003, 2(3):192-204.

[4] Hou T, Wang J, Zhang W, Xu X, ADME evaluation in drug discovery. 7. Prediction of oral absorption by correlation and classification, Journal of Chemical Information and Modeling, 2007, 47(1):208-18.

[5] Cruciani G, Carosati E, De Boeck B, Ethirajulu K, Mackie C, Howe T, Vianello R, MetaSite: understanding metabolism in human cytochromes from the perspective of the chemist, Journal of Medicinal Chemistry, 2005, 48(22):6970-9.

[6] Moroy G, Martiny VY, Vayer P, Villoutreix BO, Miteva MA, Toward *in silico* structure-based ADMET prediction in drug discovery, Drug Discovery Today. 2012,17(1-2):44-55.

[7]   Boobis A, Gundert-Remy U, Kremers P, Macheras P, Pelkonen O, *In silico* prediction of ADME and pharmacokinetics. Report of an expert meeting organised by COST B15, European Journal of Pharmaceutical Sciences, 2002, 17(4-5):183-93.

[8]   Khakar PS, Two-dimensional (2D) *in silico* models for absorption, distribution, metabolism, excretion and toxicity (ADME/T) in drug discovery, Current Topics in Medicinal Chemistry, 2010, 10(1):116-26.

[9]   Hou T, Li Y, Zhang W, Wang J, Recent developments of *in silico* predictions of intestinal absorption and oral bioavailability, Combinatorial Chemistry & High Throughput Screening, 2009, 12(5):497-506.

[10]   Kerns EH, Di L, Drug-like properties: concepts, structure, design, and methods: from ADME to toxicity optimization, 1 ed. San Diego, CA: Academic Press; 2008.

[11]   Hou T, Wang J, Zhang W, Wang W, Xu X, Recent advances in computational prediction of drug absorption and permeability in drug discovery, Current Medicinal Chemistry, 2006, 13(22):2653-67.

[12]   Egan WJ, Merz KM, Baldwin JJ, Prediction of drug absorption using multivariate statistics, Journal of Medicinal Chemistry, 2000, 19;43(21):3867-77.

[13]   Hou T, Wang J, Li Y, ADME evaluation in drug discovery. 8. The prediction of human intestinal absorption by a support vector machine, Journal of Chemical Information and Modeling, 2007, 47(6):2408-15.

[14]   Leucuta SE, Vlase L, Pharmacokinetics and metabolic drug interactions, Current Clinical Pharmacology, 2006, 1(1):5-20.

[15]   Nuez Adl, Rodríguez R, Current methodology for the assessment of ADME-Tox properties on drug candidate molecules, Biotecnología Aplicada, 2008, 25:97-110.

[16]   Lipinski CA, Lombardo F, Dominy BW, Feeney PJ, Experimental and computational approaches to estimate solubility and permeability in drug discovery and development settings Advanced Drug. Delivery Review, 2001, 46(1-3):3–26.

[17]   Chohan KK, Paine SW, Waters NJ, Advancements in Predictive *In Silico* Models for ADME, Current Chemical Biology, 2008, 2(3):215-28.

[18]   Yu LX, Lipka E, Crison JR, Amidon GL, Transport approaches to the biopharmaceutical design of oral drug delivery systems: prediction of intestinal absorption, Advanced Drug Delivery Reviews, 1996, 19(3):359-76

[19]   Kocic I, Homsek I, Dacevic M, Parojcic J, Vucicevic K, Prostran M, Miljkovic B, A case study on the *in silico* absorption simulations of levothyroxine sodium immediate-release tablets, Biopharmaceutics & Drug Disposition, 2012, 33(3):146-59.

[20]   Sinha VK, Snoeys J, Osselaer NV, Peer AV, Mackie C, Heald D, From preclinical to human – prediction of oral absorption and drug–drug interaction potential using physiologically based pharmacokinetic (PBPK) modeling approach in an industrial setting: a workflow by using case example, Biopharmaceutics & Drug Disposition, 2012, 33(2):111-21.

[21]   Grass GM, Simulation models to predict oral drug absorption from *in vitro* data, Advanced Drug Delivery Reviews, 1997, 23(1-3):199-219.

[22]   Parrott N, Lave T, Prediction of intestinal absorption: comparative assessment of GASTROPLUS (TM) and IDEA (TM), European Journal of Pharmaceutical Sciences, 2002, 17(1-2):51-61.

[23]   Testa B, Balmat A-L, Long A, Judson P, Predicting Drug Metabolism – An Evaluation of the Expert System METEOR, Chemistry & Biodiversity. 2005, 2(7):872-85.

[24]   Csete ME, Doyle JC, Reverse engineering of biological complexity, Science 2002, 295(5560):1664-9.

[25]   Tyson JJ, Chen KC, Novak B, Sniffers, buzzers, toggles and blinkers: dynamics of regulatory and signalling pathways in the cell, Current Opinion in Cell Biology, 2003, 15(2):221-31.

[26]   Wolkenhauer O, Mesarovic M, Feedback dynamics and cell function:Why systems biology is called Systems Biology, Molecular Biosystem, 2005,1(1):14-16

[27]   Ralf S, Computational approaches to the topology, stability and dynamics of metabolic networks, Phytochemistry, 2007, 68(16-18):2139-51.

[28]   Wrighton S, VandenBranden M, Ring B, The human drug metabolizing cytochromes P450, Journal of Pharmacokinetics and Pharmacodynamics, 1996, 24(5):461-73.

[29]   Nomeir AA, ADME Strategies in Lead Optimization. Early Drug Development: John Wiley & Sons, Inc.; 2010. p. 25-88.

[30]   Danielson ML, Desai PV, Mohutsky MA, Wrighton SA, Lill MA, Potentially increasing the metabolic stability of drug candidates *via* computational site of metabolism prediction by CYP2C9: The utility of incorporating protein flexibility *via* an ensemble of structures, European Journal of Medicinal Chemistry, 2011, 46(9):3953-63.

[31]   Lagorce D, Reynes C, Camproux A-C, Miteva MA, Sperandio O, Villoutreix BO, *In Silico* ADME/Tox Predictions, ADMET for Medicinal Chemists: John Wiley & Sons, Inc.; 2011. p. 29-124.

[32]   Butina D, Segall MD, Frankcombe K, Predicting ADME properties *in silico*: methods and models, Drug Discovery Today, 2002, 7(11):S83-S8.

[33]   Boulenc X, Barberan O, Metabolic-based drug-drug interactions prediction, recent approaches for risk assessment along drug development, Drug Metabolism and Drug Interaction, 2011, 26(4), 147-68.

[34]   CompuDrug International I, MetabolExpert, 115 Morgan Drive, Sedona, AZ 86351, USA2003.

[35]   Button WG, Judson PN, Long A, Vessey JD, Using absolute and relative reasoning in the prediction of the potential metabolism of xenobiotics, Journal of Chemical Information and Computer Sciences, 2003, 43(5):1371-7.

[36]   Tjollyn H, Boussery K, Mortishire-Smith RJ, Coe K, De Boeck B, Van Bocxlaer JF, Mannens G, Evaluation of three state-of-the-art metabolite prediction software packages (Meteor, MetaSite, and StarDrop) through independent and synergistic use, Durg Metabolism and Disposition, 2011, 39(11):2066-75.

[37]   Martin P, Computer-Based Methods for the Prediction of Chemical Metabolism and Biotransformation within Biological Organisms, Predicting Chemical Toxicity and Fate: CRC Press; 2004.

[38]   Benfenati E, Gini G, Computational predictive programs (expert systems) in toxicology, Toxicology, 1997, 119(3):213-25.

[39]   Smith DA, Waterbeemd Hvd, Walker DK, Pharmacokinetics and Metabolism in Drug Design. Weinheim: Wiley-VCH; 2001.

[40]   Norinder U, Bergstrom CA, Prediction of ADMET Properties, ChemMedChem, 2006, 1(9):920-37.

[41]   Wang J, Skolnik S, Recent Advances in Physicochemical and ADMET Profiling in Drug Discovery, Chemistry & Biodiversity, 2009, 6(11):1887-99.

[42] Judson R, Public Databases Supporting Computational Toxicology, Journal of Toxicology & Environmental Health: Part B, 2010, 13(2-4):218-31.

[43] Kharkar PS, Two-Dimensional (2D) *In Silico* Models for Absorption, Distribution, Metabolism, Excretion and Toxicity (ADME/T) in Drug Discovery, Current Topics in Medicinal Chemistry, 2010, 10(1):116-26.

[44] Muster W, Breidenbach A, Fischer H, Kirchner S, Muller L, Pahler A, Computational toxicology in drug development, Drug Discovery Today, 2008, 13(7-8):303-10.

[45] Valerio Jr. LG, *In silico* toxicology for the pharmaceutical sciences, Toxicology and Applied Pharmacology, 2009, 241(3):356-70.

[46] Valerio LG, Arvidson KB, Busta E, Minnier BL, Kruhlak NL, Benz RD, Testing computational toxicology models with phytochemicals, Molecular Nutrition & Food Research, 2010, 54(2):186-94.

[47] Sanderson DM, Earnshaw CG, Computer prediction of possible toxic action from chemical structure; the DEREK system, Human & Experimental Toxicology, 1991, 10(4):261-73.

[48] Ridings JE, Barratt MD, Cary R, Earnshaw CG, Eggington CE, Ellis MK, Judson PN, Langowski JJ, Marchant CA, Payne MP, Watson WP, Yih TD, Computer prediction of possible toxic action from chemical structure: an update on the DEREK system, Toxicology, 1996; 106(1-3):267-79.

[49] Mohan CG, Gandhi T, Garg D, Shinde R, Computer-assisted methods in chemical toxicity prediction. Mini Reviews in Medicinal Chemistry. 2007, 7(5):499-507.

[50] Demchuk E, Ruiz P, Wilson JD, Scinicariello F, Pohl HR, Fay M, Mumtaz MM, Hansen H, De Rosa CT, Computational toxicology methods in public health practice, Toxicology Mechanisms and Methods, 2008, 18(2-3):119-35.

[51] Lewis DF, Ioannides C, Parke DV, An improved and updated version of the compact procedure for the evaluation of P450-mediated chemical activation, Drug Metabolism Reviews, 1998, 30(4):709-37.

[52] Klopman G, Saiakhov R, Rosenkranz HS, Hermens JLM, Multiple Computer-Automated Structure Evaluation program study of aquatic toxicity 1: Guppy, Environmental Toxicology and Chemistry, 1999, 18(11):2497-505.

[53] Helma C, Lazy structure-activity relationships (lazar) for the prediction of rodent carcinogenicity and Salmonella mutagenicity, Molecular Diversity. 2006, 10(2):147-58.

[54] Gopi Mohan C, Gandhi T, Garg D, Shinde R, Computer-Assisted Methods in Chemical Toxicity Prediction, Mini Reviews in Medicinal Chemistry, 2007, 7(5):499-507.

[55] Cassano A, Manganaro A, Martin T, Young D, Piclin N, Pintore M, Bigoni D, Benfenati E. CAESAR models for developmental toxicity, Chemistry Central Journal, 2010, 4(Suppl 1):S4

[56] Frank E, Hall M, Trigg L, Holmes G, Witten IH, Data mining in bioinformatics using Weka, Bioinformatics, 2004, 20(15):2479-81.

[57] Kramer S, Raedt LD, Helma C, Molecular feature mining in HIV data. Proceedings of the seventh ACM SIGKDD international conference on Knowledge discovery and data mining; San Francisco, California. 502533: ACM; 2001. p. 136-43.

[58] Liu X, Ouyang S, Yu B, Liu Y, Huang K, Gong J,,Zheng S, Li Z, Li H, Jiang H, PharmMapper server: a web server for potential drug target identification using pharmacophore mapping approach, Nucleic Acids Research, 2010, 38:W609-14.

CHAPTER 4

Bioisosteric Replacements in Drug Design

Vinicius Barreto da Silva[1], Daniel Fábio Kawano[2], Ricardo Pereira Rodrigues[3], Susimaire Pedersoli Mantoani[3], Jonathan Resende de Almeida[3], Evandro Pizeta Semighini[3] and Carlos Henrique Tomich de Paula da Silva[3]

[1]School of Pharmaceutical Sciences of Ribeirão Preto, University of São Paulo, Ribeirão Preto, Brazil; [2]School of Pharmacy, Federal University of Rio Grande do Sul, Porto Alegre, Rio Grande do Sul, Brazil and [3]Fellow, School of Pharmaceutical Sciences of Ribeirão Preto, University of São Paulo, Ribeirão Preto, SP, Brazil

Abstract: Bioisosterism is a molecular modification Medicinal Chemistry strategy applied during drug design projects when a lead compound is available. The idea of bioisisterism is centered at the use of chemical diversity in order to optimize pharmaceutical properties of lead compounds and generate active analogs, replacing problematic substructures inside lead compounds by others with similar physicochemical properties that can improve the limitations observed for the original lead compound. Bioisosterism can be a useful strategy in order to optimize lead compounds searching for analogs with better selectivity and synthetic accessibility, decreased toxicity, improved pharmacokinetics, enhanced solubility and metabolic stability. This chapter highlights the computational approaches used to identify potential bioisosters, discusses how bioisosterism can be helpful during the design of molecules with better synthetic accessibility, and reviews the scaffold hopping technique, a novel trend of bioisosterism application intended to identify interchangeable scaffolds among pharmaceutical interesting molecules.

Keywords: Bioactivity, bioisosteric replacements, bioisosterism, chemoinformatics, drug design, drug metabolism, intermolecular interactions, lead compounds, medicinal chemistry, molecular descriptors, molecular modeling, scaffold hopping, synthetic accessibility, toxicity, virtual screening.

INTRODUCTION

Biosiosterism, term introduced by Friedman [1], can be defined as the

***Corresponding author Vinicius Barreto da Silva:** School of Pharmaceutical Sciences of Ribeirão Preto, University of São Paulo, Ribeirão Preto, Brazil; Tel: 55-62-3946-1194; E-mail: viniciusbarreto.farmacia@gmail.com

replacement of a substructure of a bioactive molecule with another substructure that is similar in size and shape and also shares physicochemical properties, having similar impact on molecular activity. Bioisosterism procedures try to maintain the biological activity of the novel chemical entity and minimize bad pharmaceutical properties related with the structure of the original query molecule. The bioisosterism term is derived from the isosteres concept, which defines group of molecules sharing the same number of atoms and valence electrons, introduced in 1919 by the physicist Irving Langmuir [2]. A broader definition of isosteres correlates molecules or substructures that have similar physicochemical properties [3-5].

Bioiosterism is a molecular modification of Medicinal Chemistry strategy applied during drug design projects when a lead compound is available [6]. The idea of bioisosterism is centered on the usage of chemical diversity in order to optimize pharmaceutical properties of lead compounds and generate active analogs, replacing problematic substructures inside lead compounds by others presenting similar physicochemical properties that can overwhelm the limitations observed for the original bioactive molecules.

The main reasons that stimulate medicinal chemists to apply bioisosterism are to optimize lead compounds, searching analogues with better selectivity, synthetic accessibility, decreased toxicity, improved pharmacokinetics, enhanced solubility and metabolic stability.

BIOSOSTERIC REPLACEMENTS

In practice, the most challenging task when performing bioiosteric replacements during drug design projects is to select or identify the most relevant interchangeable fragments in order to build novel analogues of a particular interesting lead compound. The physical and chemical properties required in a bioisosteric replacement procedure for a specific fragment in order to maintain the biological activity of a lead compound depend on which extent these properties contribute to activity and, of course, the global impact on molecular properties generated by the influence of the molecular scaffold attached to the substituted fragment [5]. Thus, suggesting appropriate bioisosteric replacements is a complex task and many molecular properties should be considered. In order to simplify this process, some strategies can be used intending to support the decision of choosing the most relevant interchangeable fragments (Fig. **1**).

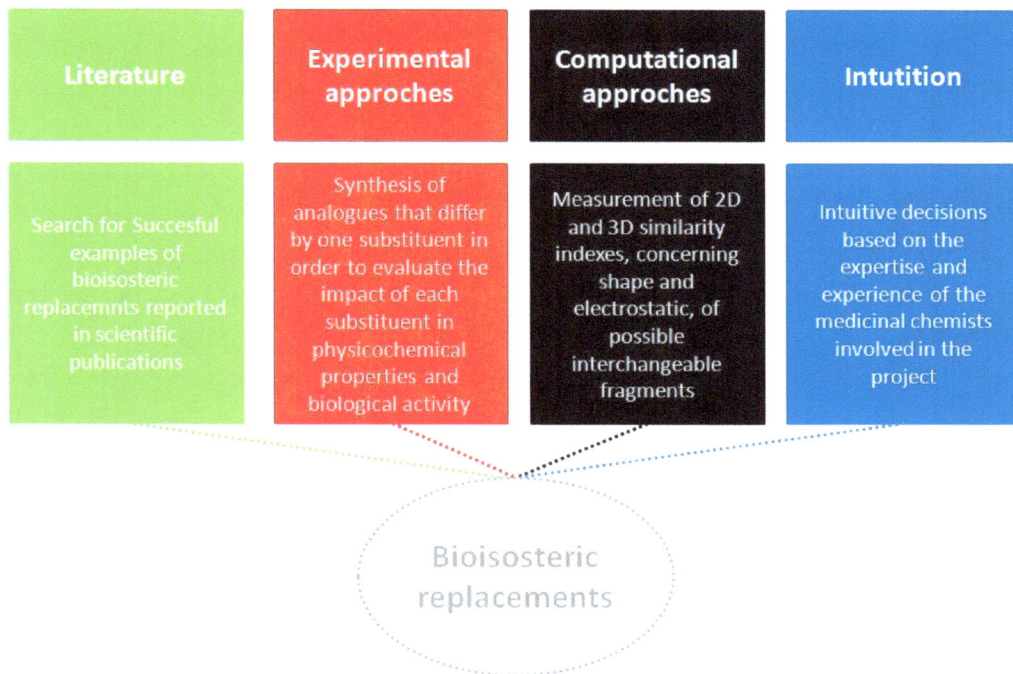

Literature	Experimental approches	Computational approches	Intuition
Search for Succesful examples of bioisosteric replacemnts reported in scientific publications	Synthesis of analogues that differ by one substituent in order to evaluate the impact of each substituent in physicochemical properties and biological activity	Measurement of 2D and 3D similarity indexes, concerning shape and electrostatic, of possible interchangeable fragments	Intuitive decisions based on the expertise and experience of the medicinal chemists involved in the project

Bioisosteric replacements

Figure 1: Kind of strategies used to identify bioisosteric replacements in Medicinal Chemistry.

One approach would be the search for successful bioisosteric replacements described in the literature. The literature search can provide a high degree of information about specific pairs of bioisosters that could be applied to novel molecular scaffolds [7]. Nevertheless, the consideration of a pair of bioisosters discovered for a specific molecular scaffold is not a guarantee of success when other different scaffolds are studied, because the structure of each novel scaffold attached to the molecular fragment will generate different molecular properties when compared with the properties observed for the original scaffold described in literature. Despite the uncertainty of the molecular properties generated by the attachment of a molecular fragment inside a new molecular scaffold, the literature search can provide an initial helpful step during bioisosteric replacement procedures in order to provide a list of possible interchangeable fragments that could be considered for initial bioisosteric replacements. Another limitation of the literature search is that the list of possible interchangeable fragments is very specific to bioisosters that had already been identified. Nevertheless, there is a need to identify novel possible bioisosteres that had not been identified in order to generate structural diversity. Performing this task, we can highlight experimental and computational approaches. During experimental approaches. the synthesis of diverse analogues of a particular molecular scaffold, limiting the variations for only one substituent, should be combined with biological evaluations in order to identify which fragments could be bioisosters of the original lead compound substituent. The major limitations of this strategy are the cost and time consumed to synthesize and evaluate an extensive series of bioactive molecules. In this way, computational approaches are extremely useful tools that can help the search for novel bioisosters [5, 8, 9] by measurements of shape and electrostatic similarity among groups of possible interchangeable fragments and guide the synthesis of novel analogues, reducing time and costs of the process where only the molecules generated by the most probable successful bioisosteric replacements are synthesized. It is important to remember that the success of a bioisosteric replacement is not centered only in maintaining biological activity but the original parameters of the lead compound should be considered which must be modified, such as toxicity, metabolic stability, solubility, synthetic accessibility and/or others.

BIOISOSTERISM AND COMPUTATIONAL APPROACHES

Appropriate bioisosteric replacement is a challenging task that requires a considerable amount of medicinal chemistry experience. Even if this experience is available, the identification of a bioisosterically suitable group with an optimal balance of steric, hydrophobic, electronic and hydrogen bonding properties usually requires an intensive procedure of trial and error. In the last years a wide range of diverse and innovative computational approaches are able to assist these replacements has been developed [5]. *In silico* methods can be very useful in the search for chemical groups sharing similar properties. These methods apply various chemoinformatic techniques based on bioactivity guided database mining, defined by the characterization of groups by a range of calculated descriptors and identification of bioisosteric pairs based on similarity of properties [3].

Since the most classical bioisosteric replacements are based on the exchange of single atoms and small groups, they are easily recognized. Nonclassical substitutions comprise less obvious exchanges, such as ring closure and ring opening, or the replacement of small substituents by larger fragments [4, 10, 11]. Therefore it is desirable to have an automated procedure to detect and assess all kinds of replacements during drug design.

The analysis of the bioisosteric fragments requires consideration of the factors affecting the ligand-target interactions, including size and shape, electronic properties (such as charge, H-bonding ability, and hidrophobicity), flexibility, and group positioning. The detailed role of these factors in ligand-protein interactions is often poorly understood, especially if there is a strong dependence on the target and ligand combination, *i.e.*, fragments found to be bioisosteric in one pair of ligands against one target may not necessarily be bioisosteric in a different pair of ligands against a different target. Such complications make the development of computational tools for the identification of bioisosteric pairs a challenging task [12]. However, several methods have been developed in order to detect a suitable replacement inside the chemical system of interest. Such tools are able to maintain key features responsible for stabilizing ligand-receptor interactions that must be present in suggested replacements, whereas features not linked to activity are assigned a lesser importance [8, 13].

Some methodologies work with the hypothesis that similarity in a selection of measured or calculated properties of a fragment will indicate a similar effect on a molecule's biological activity. These represent the first methods introduced and have as prerequisite a compact set of descriptors that, in a given context-specific information, are reliable indicators of fragment activity and are also detailed enough to filter out the many chemically similar but inactive alternatives. High computer technology enables the inclusion of more detailed information for a significant number of chemical groups, providing more accurate comparisons and reliable search results. Such rational methods are also particularly well suited to predict novel bioisosteric relationships in new and unexplored areas of the vast available chemical space [14, 15, 16].

A new and more detailed approach utilizing 3D structural information is the recently released Brood tool of OpenEye Scientific [13]. This software performs screenings in a fragment database based on steric and electrostatic similarity, allowing the user to enter a single query and perform a search in order to identify similar fragments. Each one of these fragments is further compared to the query, analyzing its three-dimensional space, chemical and electrostatic properties, and geometric arrangement of linked groups [13, 17].

Further development of rational approaches generally involves the introduction of new descriptors to act as robust indicators of similarity in fragment activity. However, descriptors for bioisosteric prediction usually need to be more general and intuitive enough to be effectively applied to a given case with only a basic understanding of what factors are important to the activity of interest. Much work has been carried out in the field of QSAR descriptor development, since it can provide 3D structural information and detailed electronic and electrostatic descriptors. [18-22].

RACHEL (*Real-time Automated Combinatorial Heuristic Enhancement of Lead compounds*) [23, 24] is an example of a different software which has implemented a computer-aided *de novo* design tool. This software was specifically designed to improve compounds with low affinity for the binding site, using an automated combinatorial method where the compounds of the database are initially divided into non rotatable groups, creating a new database. The use of models and chemical descriptors allows the program to create chemically different derivatives, increasing its ability to produce potent derivatives. To avoid the replacement of a chemical group for an inappropriate group, which could impair the receptor`s interaction, the program has an algorithm that performs the active site mapping in order to determine the chemical characteristics responsible for the receptor-ligand affinity [24].

Chemoinformatics approaches will continue to develop with the increased volume of stored data, along with the chemical diversity of compound databases. Two of the main limiting factors currently impeding the development of more reliable tools for bioisosteric prediction are the CPU cost associated with data generation for large numbers of compounds, and the efficiency and reliability of algorithms used to compare and score stored fragments to identify suitable hits. Use of more powerful machines can help address both of these issues, and is likely to lead to the development of more ambitious and reliable tools in the future. The ability of algorithms to predict suitable hits might be improved by the incorporation of available binding site information, and by the use of machine learning techniques to help characterize the origins of fragment activity. Such approaches are becoming more common in the related field of the *de novo* fragment drug design [25].

As computational methods for bioisosteric prediction become more accepted and reliable, their application to lead optimization problems will become increasingly widespread. The ultimate measure of the benefit brought by each method will be its ability to help chemists to make effective structural modifications quickly, and to offer an increased diversity of chemical substituents by making novel predictions that can complement the safer selection of known transformations that are currently in use [5].

SCAFFOLD HOPPING

Scaffold hopping is a technique closely related to the prediction of bioisosterism. Both scaffold hopping method and the bioisosteric replacement are used to improve synthetic accessibility, potency and drug-like properties of an active compound, as well as joining a new chemical space. The main idea of this approach is to create new chemical entities by keeping a sufficient similarity with the originalbioactive compound in order to maintain the biological activity after changing the core of the compound and moving it to a new chemical space [3]. Scaffold hopping can be defined as a method used to discover new chemical classes by replacing a part (scaffold, the core of the molecule) of a known compound preserving the remaining chemical groups under the assumption that they are important to biological activity [26].

Therefore, the challenge of scaffold hopping is to identify molecular cores which will form the mainstay of new families of compounds with similar biological activity to a known reference molecule. This goal is reached when through the search of scaffolds, the relative group orientations that interact directly with the target binding site are kept functional [5]. This prevents not only problems with intellectual property rights but also allows the exploration of new and potentially much more interesting scaffolds that fulfill the same role of the reference active molecules. Thus, scaffold hopping refers to the identification of different classes of compounds having similar biological activity. In Medicinal Chemistry, the search for different structural classes with similar biological activity is of high interest in virtual screening methods [27].

One example of successful application of scaffold hopping is reported by Tung *et al* [28], where the replacement of the indole ring of a potent anticancer agent, targeting tubulin, by alternative 5,6-fused bicyclic heteroaromatics helped the design of novel drug candidates with new intellectual property rights (Fig. **2**). Compounds A, B and C docked to the colchicine binding site in a similar way to that of the indole scaffold, suggesting an antiproliferative mechanism similar with the observed for the indole lead compound. Most interestingly, compound C, an orally bioavailable anticancer agent, showed improved metabolic stability and better aqueous solubility than the original indole lead compound.

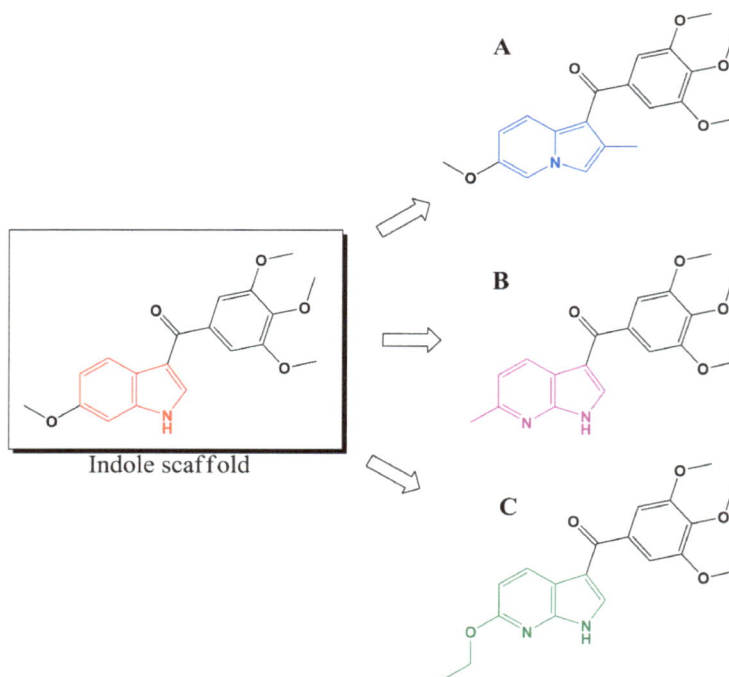

Figure 2: Application of a scaffold hopping procedure, where the indolic scaffold of the original reference molecule is substituted for new 5,6-fused bicyclic heteroaromatics [28].

There are many available methods for *in silico* bioisosteric replacements and scaffold hopping to identify groups with similar properties. These methods apply various techniques of chemoinformatics as the characterization of groups by a large number of calculated descriptors and identification of bioisosteric pairs based on similarity of properties. Langdon *et al.* [3] report different types of descriptors that have been described and compiling distinct molecular properties for different applications. These descriptors can be grouped into three main categories: topological descriptors (2D descriptors that retain information on molecular characteristics such as atoms, types of atoms, substructures, and how these characteristics are connected with the molecules), topographic descriptors (also descriptors of molecular characteristics, but retain information from geometric of these features and are, thus, 3D descriptors) and surface-based or field-based descriptors (are also 3D descriptors, but encode information on the surface of the molecule or molecular field).

Bergmann and coworkers [29] presented a GRID-based method for scaffold hopping, the SHOP methodology. This similarity search approach based on GRID identifies new scaffolds in a database by analyzing the similarity of their three-dimensional structures with those query scaffolds. The aim of such approach is to find substituents for consulting the scaffold while the geometry, form and patterns of interaction of the central fragment of the query ligand are retained. For this, the descriptors used for these searches are specific anchor points, where the anchor refers to positions on the scaffolds. In the SHOP software, scaffolds are described geometrically in accordance with the distance and dihedral angles between their anchor points. The scaffold's shape is based on analysis of these distances between each anchor point and the surface of the scaffold calculated with MIFs. The GRID program is then used to obtain the description of the scaffold's shape by calculating the energies of the interaction in a grid-shaped box around the scaffold, thus, obtaining the distances between each anchor point and each grid point with an energy value that is registered. The most favorable energy values are selected. These anchor points selected are then used in the search step within molecular databases by similarity. Thus, with the scaffolds selected within the database it is possible to create new scaffolds which are able to retain the desired ligand properties of the original bioactive scaffold.

Rush *et al* [30] described the first application of ROCS (Rapid Overlay of Chemical Structures, an OpenEye Scientific Software) in order to find new scaffolds for small molecular inhibitors of an antibacterial target. This implemented method for scaffold hopping uses an algorithm that finds the greatest amount of overlap between two 3D molecules. It is based on the entire volume of the molecule and not only on the surface. The emphasis and purpose of this approach is to identify molecules from databases that can adopt very similar shapes to the query molecules, thus, increasing chances of scaffold hopping. The database used contain molecules with molecular weights between 180 and 400 Da, less than nine rotatable bonds, molecules with only one chiral center, logD lower than 4 and less than 4 ionizable groups. These molecules were increased to a set of 3D conformers using the OMEGA software. Thus, two new scaffolds were found and they were significantly different for the proposed target using this algorithm. The active compounds were identified without any reference to the chemistry details of known active compounds. The ROCS approach is based on an intuitive fragmentation based on physicochemical reasoning of the known active compounds to generate appropriate models for the searches. This is what differs from other 3D search methods. The experimental results presented in this study validated the use of ROCS for scaffold hopping, and suggest that its application for the purpose of identifying new compounds is of great interest in drug discovery.

As one of the main tools used for scaffold hopping, virtual screening has received widespread attention because it is a technique often used in drug discovery programs. For this, a screening is performed in a large database of potential compounds for drug candidates targeting a protein or a reference molecule to subsequently select a subset of compounds for experimental testing. For the prominence of virtual screening methods to successfully run scaffold hopping, many descriptors have been developed to measure its effectiveness [31].

A complementary program to the ROCS program is EON (an OpenEye Scientific Software) for electrostatic potential calculations. EON is a descriptor used for scaffold hopping, it calculates the similarity of two pre-aligned molecules based on their electrostatic fields. That is, the overlaps and alignments of pairs of molecular structures made by ROCS, EON calculates the electrostatic field around each of the molecules using ZAP toolkit, a solver of the Poisson-Boltzmann equation [19]. López-Ramos & Perruccio [31] described the use of this tool as a ligand-based and target-based virtual screening. In this study, both virtual screening and scaffold hopping methods were evaluated. The protein chosen was hidroxyphenilpyruvatedioxigenase (HPPD) which is involved in the tyrosine degradation pathway and thus, HPPD is a target for the treatment of hypertyrosinemia in humans. In plants, this is an important enzyme for plastoquinone and tocopherol production. Inhibition of this enzyme causes a bleaching, followed by necrosis and death of the plant. The HPPD inhibitors have generated a considerable number of herbicides which are marketed stemming from research carried out in the agrochemical industries. The ligand mesotrione (Fig. **3**) is the main representative of such an herbicides chemical class. Although the methods of virtual screening (lead finding and scaffold hopping) are mostly associated with the pharmaceutical context, in the agrochemical area the fundamental concept of this approach remains the same as in drug discovery.

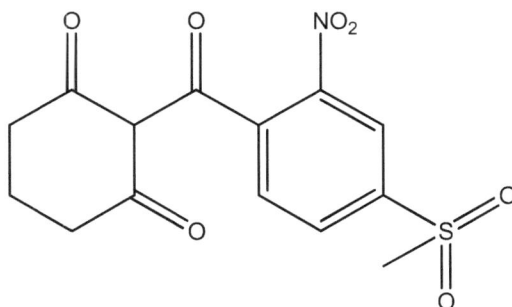

Figure 3: Chemical structure of mesotrione.

Examples from literature have shown the importance of the scaffold hopping approach and its successful application. In the discovery of novel cannabinoid 1 (CB$_1$) receptor, Boström *et al.* [32] demonstrate the concept of scaffold hopping in Rimonabant (Acomplia^{TM}), a CB$_1$ receptor antagonist for the treatment of obesity. In order to improve physicochemical and pharmacodynamics properties, a scaffold hopping approach was applied for altering the central fragment, the methylpyrazole, in Rimonabant. This work described the design of a new series of 5,6-diaryl-pyrazine-2-amide derivatives and many of these compounds showed IC$_{50}$ values below 10 nM for the CB$_1$ receptor (Fig. **4**).

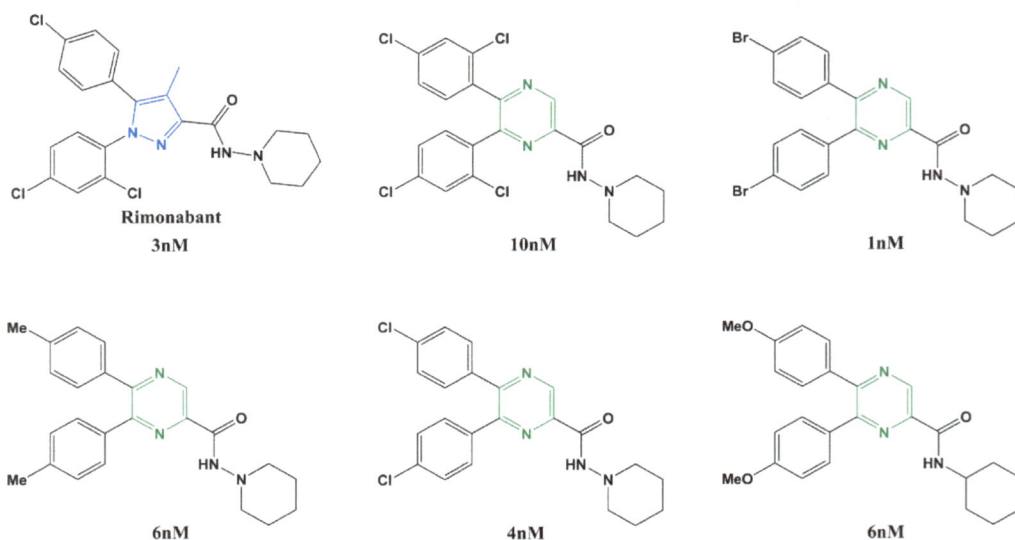

Figure 4: Structure and IC_{50} values for compounds with *N*-piperidylamide substituents. The IC_{50} are presented for the CB1 antagonists with *in vitro* potency below 10nM.

Another interesting example is the application of the scaffold hopping approach in the discovery of a novel indole series of EP_1 receptor antagonist as potential analgesics [33]. The authors proposed the design of novel EP_1 receptor antagonists for the treatment of inflammatory pain based on the concept that the new template would have an improvement in potency, selectivity and/or pharmacokinetics over the starting template. Stimulated by their previous reported results regarding the pyrazole, thiazole and pyridine derivatives and intrigued by the potential hydrogen bond formed between the *ortho*-alkoxy group and the biaryl NH of a generic structure (Fig. **5A**), they synthesized a series of indole compounds of general structure B (Fig. **5B**).

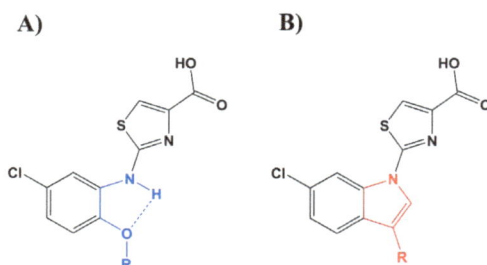

Figure 5: (**A**) Potential intramolecular bond that could be formed between the ortho-alkoxy group, and (**B**) the biaryl NH of a generic structure.

The compounds prepared (Fig. **6**) and tested proved to be potent EP_1 receptor antagonists. For the compound where R was i-Bu, the result presented was binding pIC_{50} of 8.2 and a pKi of 9.3±0.3 in a functional assay. The SAR also showed that large groups (CH_2CH_2t-Bu) are the best choice.

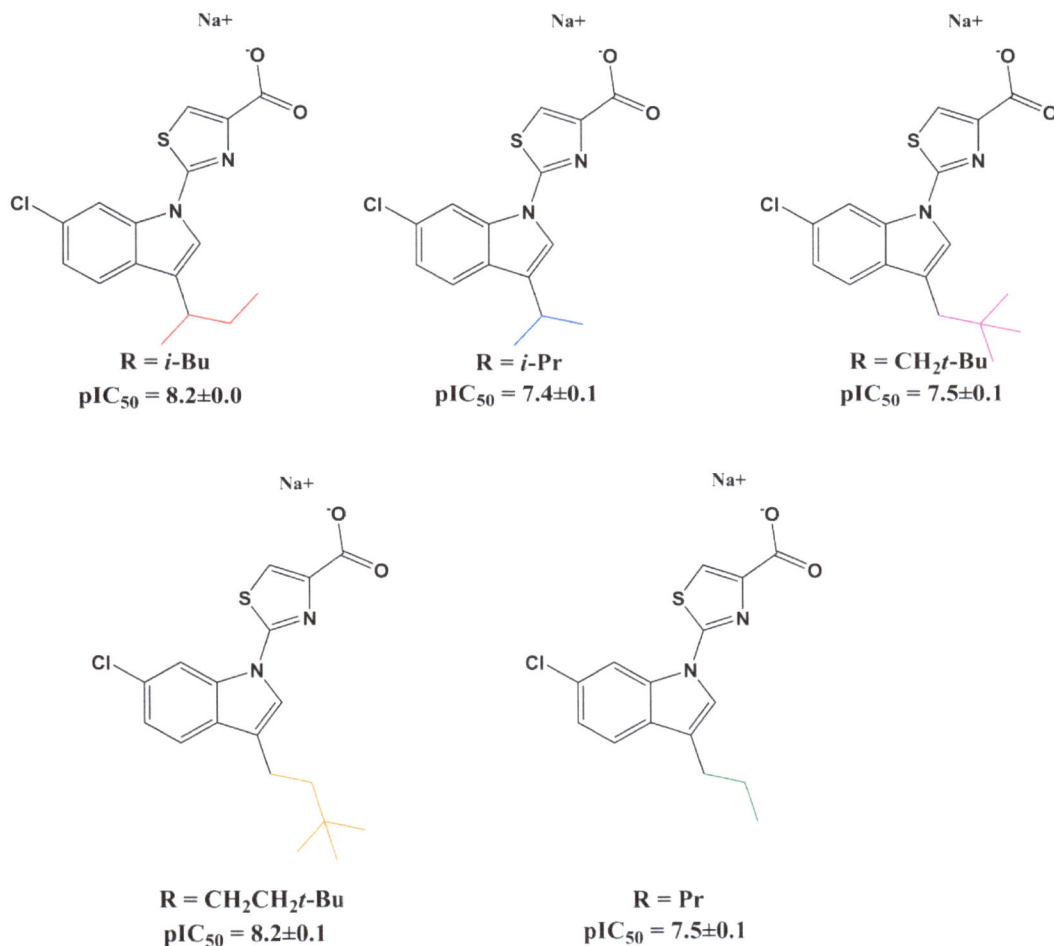

Figure 6: SAR for the EP_1 receptor antagonists proposed by Hall *et al*. [33].

BIOISOSTERIC REPLACEMENTS AS A STRATEGY TO IMPROVE SYNTHETIC ACCESSIBILITY

Chemical synthesis is an important issue and often a limiting factor in the drug discovery process [34]. Although bioinformatics, chemoinformatics and theoretical drug optimization strategies are valuable and integral parts of the drug design process, they may sometimes generate structures that are quite complicated and, consequently, hard to synthesize by requiring long-step synthesis with carefully controlled reactions, especially if the stereochemical configuration is a concern [35]. Therefore, the factors that contribute to make a synthesis difficult to execute (*i.e.* those which give rise to molecular complexity) [36] must be considered when selecting a hit or preparing analogs for a hit of interest.

Medicinal chemists typically aim to synthesize as many new compounds as quickly as possible which can then be tested by biologists against a chosen biological target [37]. In this context, synthetic accessibility can be considered as an effort to use the smallest number of chemical steps to synthesize a drug from common laboratory reactants [38]. However, synthetic accessibility and structural complexity are not only central issues in determining potential drug candidate molecules. They also must be carefully analyzed in the subsequent creation, exploration, and evaluation of short, efficient, safe, reproducible, scalable, ecological but still economical synthesis for the selected clinical candidates, *i.e.* in process optimization and scale up synthesis [37].

From the structural point of view, several features contribute to molecular complexity such as molecular size, element and functional-group content, cyclic connectivity, stereocenter content, chemical reactivity and structural instability [36]. Although these factors had been primarily identified based on the experience of organic chemists regarding what features in the structure of a compound make it hard to be synthesized, there are also theoretical reasons for recognizing some of these features as sources of complexity. As stated by Goodwin [39] "the more functional groups a structure has, the more likely it is that one of those functional groups will interfere with an attempt to apply a standard chemical reaction to modify a structure in a predictable way. Similarly, the more structurally unstable a molecule is, the more likely an attempted chemical modification of it will result in a range of possible products. Not only are reagents often capable of reacting at multiple sites in a complex molecule, but also structural complexity can alter the chemical environment in a way that interferes with the mechanism of a desired reaction so that it will no longer produce the desired product to the anticipated extent."

Though bioisosteres are classically used by medicinal chemists to improve potency, selectivity, bioavailability and/or metabolic stability, to decrease side effects or even to achieve patentability. Bioisteric replacements can also result in compounds with reduced structural complexity and, consequently, better synthetic accessibility. This can be achieved by improving structural stability, for example, when an ester group is replaced by an amide (Fig. **7**), which is more resistant to chemical hydrolysis, or when a methyl group of an ethanoate ester is replaced with NH_2 (Fig. **4**), thus generating an urethane functional group [40].

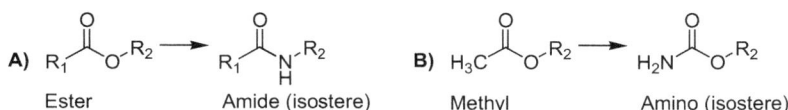

Figure 7: Isosteric replacement of (**A**) an ester with an amide and (**B**) a methyl with an amino group.

Bioisosterism also can be helpful to adapt the structure of a compound to a more feasible or commercially convenient synthesis. In the synthesis of pteridine analogues designed as anticancer agents, the authors synthesized analogue **I** in three steps from commercial 2,4-dihydroxy-5,6-diaminopyrimidine (Fig. **8**). To obtain its bioisostericsurrogate**II** (that in fact proved to be more active than **I** itself), the synthesis was accomplished in only one step starting from commercially available 2,4-diamino-6,7-dimethylpteridine [41].

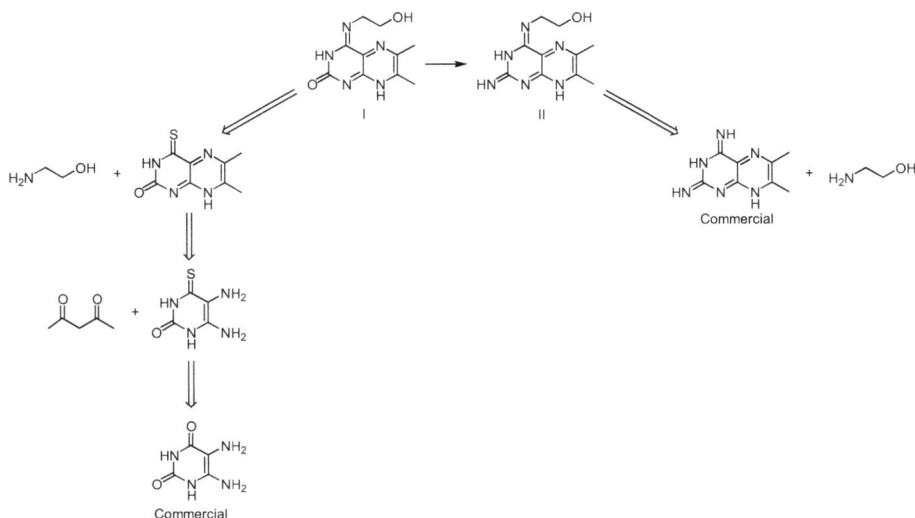

Figure 8: Syntheses of pteridine analogues designed as anticancer agents [41].

Based on studies that identified the triazole ring as a starting point for the design of oxytocin antagonists, Brown *et al.* [42, 43] synthesized a series of potent, selective and orally-bioavailable compounds with the ability to antagonize the physiological effects of oxytocin. Subsequently, the authors synthesized amide bioisosteres of the previously reported triazoleoxytocin antagonists and the higher synthetic accessibility of the amides (Fig. **9**) allowed the utilization of synthetic libraries to find new substituents for design of novel lead compounds [42, 43].

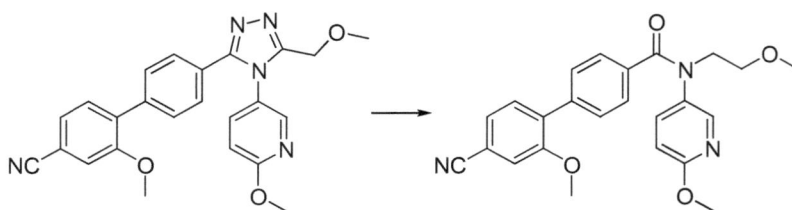

Figure 9: A triazole oxytocin antagonist and its amide bioisoster [42, 43].

Another interesting case that illustrates how bioisosteres can improve synthetic accessibility refers to the development of the antidepressant agomelatine, which is a synthetic melatonin analog that acts as agonist at melatonergic MT_1 and MT_2 receptors and antagonist at serotonin $5HT_{2C}$ receptors [44]. Although agomelatine can be considered slightly less potent than melatonin [45], the replacement of the isoindole ring of melatonin (Fig. **10**) by a naphthalene ring in agomelatine (Fig. **11**) resulted in considerably simplification in the industrial preparation of the antidepressant.

In the industrial synthesis of melatonin (Fig. **10**), the primary alkyl halide 1-bromo-3-chloropropane is converted into a primary amine *via* N-alkylatation of phthalimide followed by amine deprotection by acid hydrolysis, a process known as Gabriel synthesis. The isoindole ring is generated in multiple steps by converting the N-(3-chloropropyl)phthalimide to N-(3-iodopropyl)phthalimide in the presence of sodium iodide, condensing the N-(3-iodopropyl)phthalimide with ethyl 3-oxobutanoate in the presence of a base and reacting the corresponding product with a diazonium salt of *p*-anisidine to form the indole derivative. Melatonin is then generated by decarboxylation and acetylation of the 5-methoxy tryptamine.

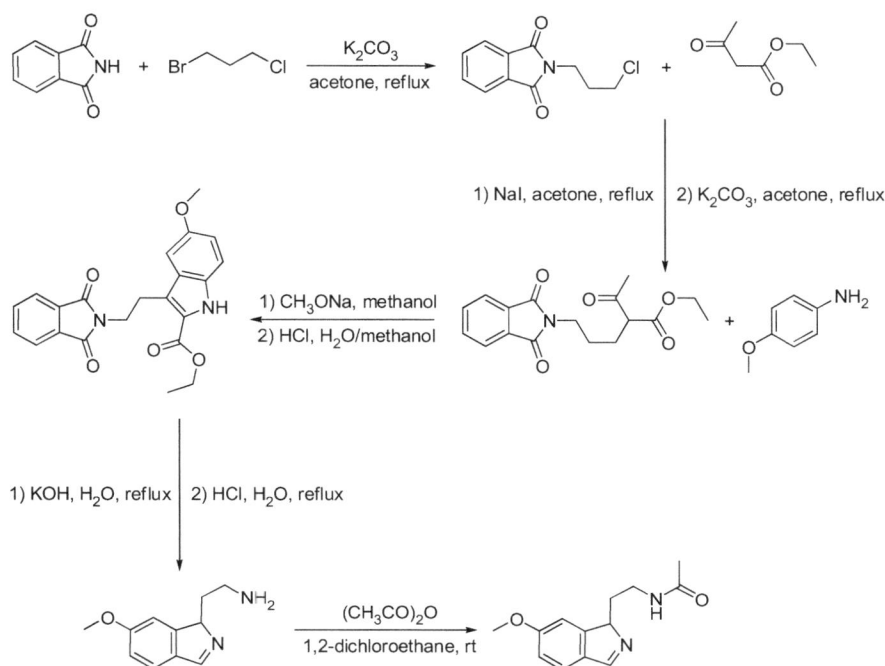

Figure 10: Synthesis of melatonin [46].

The replacement of the isoindole ring by a naphthalene ring, allowed the design of the industrial synthesis of agomelatine starting from the commercial reagent 7-methoxy-1-tetralone (Fig. **11**). In this process, the cyclohexanone group of 7-methoxy-1-tetralone is converted into a nitrile derivative using cyanoacetic acid (Fig. **11**, Step 1), aromatized *via* palladium on carbon catalysis (Fig. **11**, Step 2) followed by the reduction of the nitrile to amine (Fig. **11**, Step 3) and acetylation (Fig. **11**, Step 4) to give agomelatine.

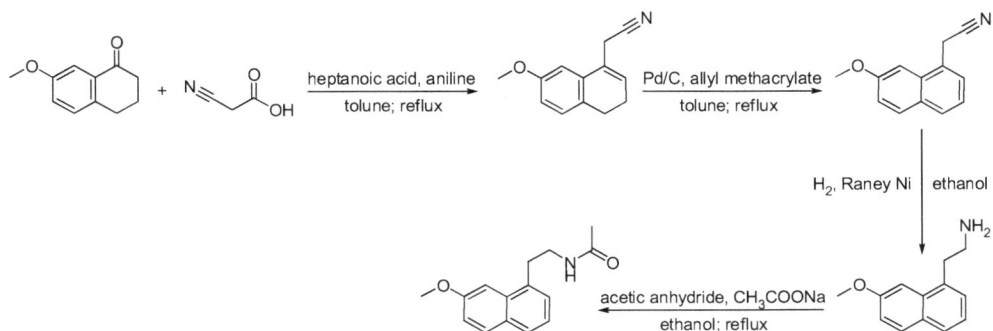

Figure 11: Synthesis of melatonin [47].

SUCCESSFUL EXAMPLES OF BIOISOSTERIC REPLACEMENTS IN DRUG DESIGN

There are innumerous examples of successful drugs already introduced in the clinical practice that are derivatives of other drugs or bioactive molecules, where the implementation of bioisosteric replacements were a key step during their design. One example is the development of clorpropamide from tolbutamide, where the change of only one substituent led to a drug with better pharmaceutical profile. Tolbutamide (Fig. **12**) is a first generation potassium channel blocker that stimulates the secretion of insulin by the pancreas and is used in the treatment of type II diabetes. Tolbutamide has a short time of action due to the fast metabolism of the benzilic carbon of its structure. This led to the development of clorpropramide (Fig. **12**), a tolbutamide derivative, where the methyl radical of the aromatic ring was substituted by a chlorine, thus avoiding the CYP-450 oxidation of this methyl and making the Clorpropramide a drug with prolonged time of action [40, 48].

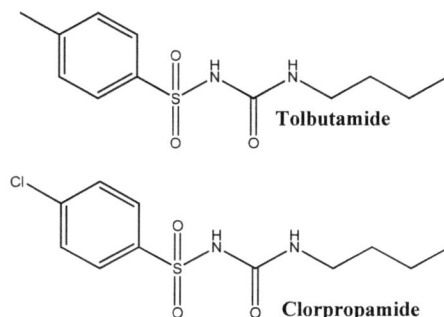

Figure 12: Structures of potassium channel blockers Tolbutamide and Clorpropramide.

Celecoxib (Fig. **13**) was the first anti-inflammatory drug with selective inhibitory activity over COX-2 (cycloxigenase-2). It has low penetration on the BBB (Brain Blood Barrier), presenting a Brain/Plasma ratio of 0.1 and, consequently, low activity in inflammatory processes on the central nervous system (CNS). The Brain/Plasma ratio is improved to 0.8 mainly by the introduction of a methyl sulfone on Refecoxib (Fig. **13**), a less polar bioisoster of the original sulfonamide present at celecoxib, allowing a higher penetration trough the BBB and a better activity against inflammatory processes in the CNS [49].

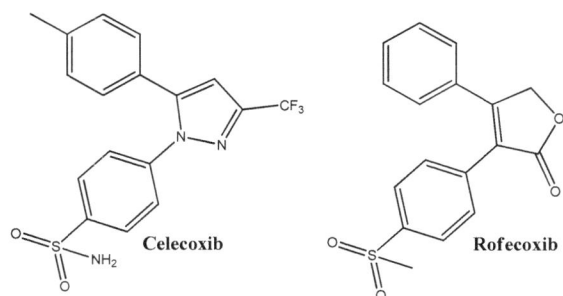

Figure 13: Structures of selective COX-2 Inhibitors Celecoxib and Rofecoxib.

Procaine (Fig. **14**) was one of the first anesthetics synthesized by man and was widely used in clinical until the introduction of more effective alternatives like lidocaine (Fig. **14**). Procaine has a vasodilator effect and is often co administered with a vasoconstrictor, like adrenaline, to reduce the bleeding and the clearance of procaine of the local where it was injected. Procaine has an ester on its structure and it's hydrolyzed in the plasma by the enzyme pseudocholinesterase, making it a lasting drug. To avoid this hydrolysis, the ester was changed by an isosteric amide and there are two *orto*-methyl groups in the aromatic ring, creating a steric shield to the amide, leading to Lidocaine, a longer acting local anesthetic [40, 49, 50].

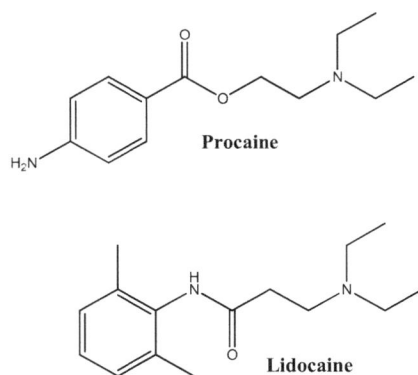

Figure 14: Structures of local anesthetics Procaine and Lidocaine.

Nifedipine (Fig. **15**) is a calcium-channel antagonist administered orally in the treatment of hipertension, despite its low bioavailability due to reduced hidrosolubilityand the quick metabolic reduction of the aromatic nitro group. Nifedipine is often formulated with polyvinylpyrrolidone (PVP) and polyethyleneglycols (PEG) for a better dissolution and absorption by the gut wall.

Felodipine (Fig. **15**) uses bioisosteric substitution of the nitrobenzene group by a dichlorobenzene to have better hidrosolubility and improved half-life, from 2 to 17 hours when compared with nidefipine, by avoiding the metabolic reduction observed by the nitro group [49].

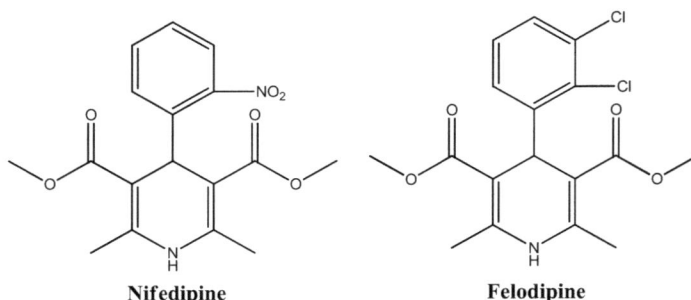

Nifedipine   Felodipine

Figure 15: Structures of Calcium Channel Antagonists Nifedipine and Felodipine.

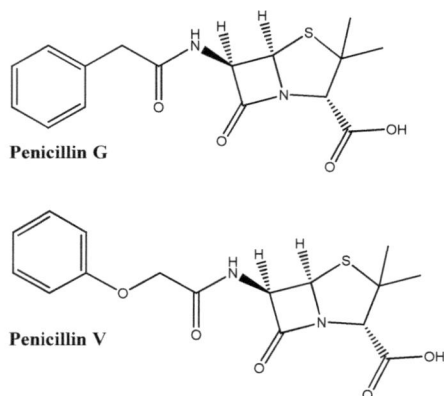

Figure 16: Structures of beta-lactamic antibiotics Penicillin G and Penicillin V.

Penicillin G (Fig. **16**) was the first antibiotic drug widely used by mankind, but due to the high susceptibility of the beta-lactamic ring of its structure by acid hydrolysis, it must be injected by intramuscular or intravenous ways to avoid degradation by the gastric acid.The beta-lactamic ring is essential for the mechanism of action of all penicillins, but the ring tension makes the carbonyl of the beta-lactam more eletrophilic than other amides due to the lack of a dipolar resonance between the carbonyl and the nitrogen that normally exists in amide systems, this makes the beta-lactamic ring more susceptible to the attack of a nucleophile, causing the acid sensitivity of the Penicillin G. In order to reduce this acid sensibility, the phenoxymetyl group, a more electron-withdrawing isoster than the benzyl group, is used in Penicillin V (Fig. **16**), reducing the nucleophilicity of the carbonyl and, consequently, its susceptibility to the acid attack, allowing the Penicillin V to be taken orally [40].

Another approach already used in penicillins is the change or modification of the benzilic system by a bulkier group to avoid the enzimatic beta lactamase degradation induced for some bacteria as an antibiotic resistance mechanism. Nafcillin and oxacillin (Fig. **17**) are interesting examples of beta-lactamic drugs with bulkier groups acting as steric shields, making them resistant to bacterial beta-lactamases [40].

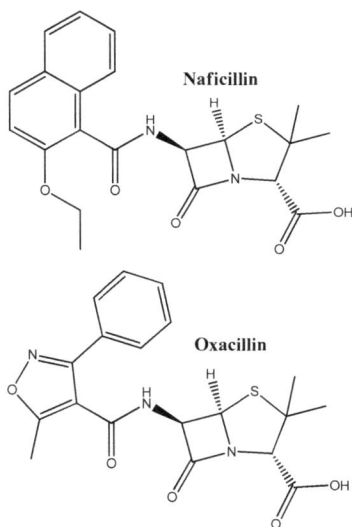

Figure 17: Structures of beta-lactamic antibiotics Nafcillin and Oxacillin.

Burimamide (Fig. **18**) is a compound developed as a histamine H2-receptor antagonist to the treatment of gastric ulcer. Despite the good inhibitory activity, it's not absorbed by the gut wall and lacks oral bioavailability. This stimulated the development of methiamide (Fig. **18**) by adding a methyl group in the position 4 of the imidazolic ring and the change of a carbon atom by a sulfur atom in the side chain, reducing the ionization of the imidazol ring and giving methiamide a good oral bioavailability and 10 times more potency. Unfortunately, the metabolism of the thiourea group causes toxicity and methiamide wasn't approved in phase I

Clinical Trials. The isosteric substitution of the tiourea by an N-cianoguanidine led the synthesis of cimetidine (Fig. **18**), the first anti gastric ulcer drug to hit the market, keeping the activity and bioavailability of methiamide without its severe toxic effects [40, 49].

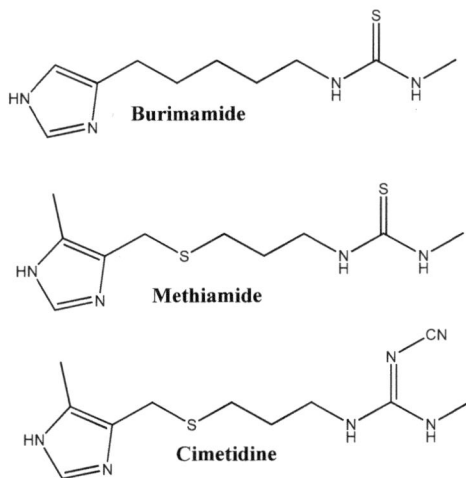

Figure 18: Chemical structures of Burimamide, Methiamide and Cimetidine.

CONCLUSION

The bioisosteric replacement strategy can be very useful in many ways during drug properties optimization, including the design of penicillins that can be taken orally, the design of novel calcium channel antagonists with increased half-life and the synthesis of antidepressants with simplified industrial preparation. Such chemical optimizations are driven by the knowledge created over many years of Medicinal Chemists experience during the design of several drugs in the modern era. However, there is a need for rationalizing this task and identifying useful bioisosteric replacements faster, reducing time and costs. In this scenario, we can verify that many scientific groups are using chemical databases and molecular descriptors knowledge trying to achieve the development of reliable chemoinformatic approaches able to identify structural similarities among groups of molecular fragments. This will make bioisosteric replacements an easier task and help chemists to make effective structural modifications quickly during the different drug design steps.

ACKNOWLEDGEMENTS

We acknowledge financial support from CNPq and FAPESP.

CONFLICT OF INTEREST

The authors confirm that this chapter contents have no conflict of interest.

REFERENCES

[1]　Friedman HL. Influence of isosteric replacements upon biological activity. Symposium on Chemical-Biological Correlation.National Research Council Publication, Washington, EUA,1951, n 206, p. 295.

[2]　Langmuir I. Isomorphism, isosterism and covalence. Journal of the American Chemical Society, 1959, 41: 1543-1559.

[3]　Langdon SR, Ertl P, Brown N. Bioisosteric replacements and scaffold hopping in lead generation and optimization. Molecular Informatics, 2010, 29: 366-385.

[4]　Lima LM, Barreiro EJ. Bioisosterism: a useful strategy for molecular modification and drug design. Current Medicinal Chemistry, 2005, 12: 23-49.

[5]　Devereux M, Popelier PLA. *In silico* techniques for the identification of bioisosteric replacements for drug design. Current Topics in Medicinal Chemistry, 2010, 10:657-668.

[6]　Bhatia R, SharmaV, Shrivastava, Singla RK. A review on bioisosterism: a rational approach for drug design and molecular modification. Pharmacologyonline, 2011,1:272-299, 2011.

[7]　Meanwell NA. Synopsis of some recent tactical applications of bioisosters in drug design. Journal of Medicinal Chemistry, 2011, 54: 2529-2591.

[8]　Devereux M, Popelier PLA, Mclay IM. Quantum isosteredatabase : a web-based tool using quantum chemical topology to predict bioisosteric replacements for drug design. Journal of Chemical Information and Modeling, 2009, 49:1497-1513.

[9]　Wagener M, Lommerse JPM. The quest for bioisosteric replacements. Journal of Chemical Information and Modeling, 2006, 46:677-685.

[10]　Patani GA, Lavoie EJ. Bioisosterism: A Rational Approach in Drug Design. Chemical Reviews, 1996, 96:3147–3176.

[11]　Krier M, Hutter MC. Bioisosteric Similarity of Molecules Based on Structural Alignment and Observed Chemical Replacements in Drugs. Journal of Chemical Information and Modeling, 2009, 49:1280-1297.

[12]　Birchall K, Gillet VJ, Willett P. Use of Reduced Graphs To Encode Bioisosterism for Similarity-Based Virtual Screening. Journal of Chemical Information and Modeling, 2009, 49: 1330-1346.

[13]　BROOD. Fragment replacement for Medicinal Chemistry. version 1.1.2. Santa Fe, New Mexico: OpenEye Scientific Software, 2009.

[14]　Ertl P. Cheminformatics analysis of organic substituents: identification of the most common substituents, calculation of substituent properties, and automatic identification of

drug-like bioisosteric groups. Journal of Chemical Information and Computer Sciences, 2003, 43:374-380.

[15] Bohacek RS, McMartin C, Guida WC. The art and practice of structure-based drug design: A molecular modeling perspective. Medicinal Research Reviews,1996,16:03-50.

[16] Weininger D. In: *Encyclopedia of Computational Chemistry*; Schleyer PVR, Allinger N L, Clark T, Gasteiger J, Kollman PA, Schaefer III HF, Schreiner PR. Eds.; John Wiley & Sons: Chichester, UK, 1998,1: 425-430.

[17] Corkery JJ, Skillman AG, Schmidt KE, Kelley B. Visualization and analysis of bioisosteric analogs generated with BROOD. In: 239th ACS National Meeting, 2010, San Francisco, CA, United States. Proceedings. American Chemical Society.

[18] Popelier PLA, Smith PJ. QSAR models based on quantum topological molecular similarity. European Journal of Medicinal Chemistry, 2006, 41: 862-873.

[19] Nicholls A, Maccuish NE, Maccuish JD. Variable selection and model validation of 2D and 3D molecular descriptors. Journal of Computer-Aided Molecular Design, 2004, 18:7-9.

[20] Hopfinger AJ, Wang S, Tokarsk JS, Jin BQ, Albuquerque M, Madhav PJ, Duraiswam C. Construction of 3D-QSAR models using the 4D-QSAR analysis formalism. Journal of the American Chemical Society, 1997, 119:10509-10524.

[21] Pastor M, Cruciani G, Mclay I, Pickett S, Clementi S. GRid-INdependent descriptors (GRIND): A novel class of alignment independent three-dimensional molecular descriptors. Journal of Medicinal Chemistry,2000, 43:3233-3243.

[22] Silverman BD, Platt DE. Comparative molecular moment analysis (CoMMA): 3D-QSAR without molecular superposition. Journal of Medicinal Chemistry, 1996, 39:2129-2140.

[23] Oprea TI. (Ed). Chemoinformatics in Drug Discovery. Methods and Principles in Medicinal Chemistry: WILEY-VCH, v.23, p.490, Methods and Principles in Medicinal Chemistryed. 2005.

[24] SYBYL. SYBYL-X 1.2, Tripos International, 1699 South Hanley Rd., St. Louis, Missouri, 63144, USA. 2010.

[25] Nicolaou CA, Apostlolakis J, Pattichis, C. S. *De novo* drug design using multiobjective evolutionary graphs. Journal of Chemical Information and Modeling, 2009, 49:295-307.

[26] Deschênes A, Sourial E. Ligand Scaffold replacement using MOE pharmacophore tools. Chemical Computing Group Inc., 2007. Avaliable at: http://www.chemcomp.com/journal/scaffold.htm

[27] Hu Y, Bajorath J. Global assessment of scaffold hopping potential for current pharmaceutical targets. Medchemcomm, 2010,1: 339-344.

[28] Tung YS, Coumar MS, Wu YS, Shiao HY, Chang JY, Liou JP, Shukla P, Chang CW, Chang CY, Ku CC, Yeh TK, Lin CY, Wu JS, Wu SY, Liao CC, Hsieh HP. Scaffold-hopping strategy: synthesis and biological evaluation of 5,6-fused bicyclic heteroaromatics to identify orally bioavailable anticancer agents. Journal of Medicinal Chemistry, 2011, 54:3076-3080.

[29] Bergmann R.; Linusson A. Zamora I. SHOP: Scaffold HOPping by GRID-based similarity searches. Journal of Medicinal Chemistry, 2007, 50: 2708-2717.

[30] Rush TS, Grant JA, Mosyak L, Nicholls A. A shape-based 3-D scaffold hopping method and its application to a bacterial protein-protein interaction. Journal of Medicinal Chemistry, 2005, 48: 1489-1495.

[31] Lopez-Ramos M, Perruccio F. HPPD: ligand- and target-based virtual screening on a herbicide target. Journal of Chemical Information and Modeling, 2010,50:801-814.

[32]   Boström J, Berggren K, Elebring T, Greasley PJ, Wilstermann M. Scaffold hopping, synthesis and structure-activity relationships of 5,6-diaryl-pyrazine-2-amide derivatives: a novel series of CB1 receptor antagonists. Bioorganic & Medicinal Chemistry, 2007, 15:4077-4084.

[33]   Hall A, Billinton A, Brown SH, Chowdhury A, Giblin GM, Goldsmith P, Hurst DN, Naylor A, Patel S, Scoccitti T, Theobald PJ. Discovery of a novel indole series of EP1 receptor antagonists by scaffold hopping. Bioorganic & Medicinal Chemistry Letters, 2008, 18: 2684-2690.

[34]   Schurer SC, Tyagi P, Muskal SM. Prospective exploration of synthetically feasible, medicinally relevant chemical space. Journal of Chemical Information and Modeling, 2005, 45: 239-248.

[35]   Gasteiger J. *De novo* design and synthetic accessibility. Journal of Computer-Aided Molecular Design, 2007, 21:307-309, 2007.

[36]   Corey EJ, Chelg XM. The logic of chemical synthesis. 1st ed. New York: John Wiley, 1995. 436 p.

[37]   Karpf M. From milligrams to tons: the importance of synthesis and process research in the development of new drugs. In: Shioiri T, Izawa K, Konoike T. (Ed). Pharmaceutical process chemistry. 1st ed. New York: WILEY-VCH Verlag GmbH & Co, 2011. Chapter 1, p. 01-38.

[38]   Wunderlich Z, Mirny LA. Using the topology of metabolic networks to predict viability of mutant strains. Biophysical Journal, 2006, 91:2304-2311.

[39]   Goodwin W. Scientific understanding and synthetic design. British Journal for the Philosophy of Science, 2009, 60 271-301.

[40]   Patrick GL. An introduction to medicinal chemistry. 4th ed. Oxford: Oxford University Press, 2009.

[41]   Chauhan PMS, Martins CJA, Horwell DC. Syntheses of novel heterocycles as anticancer agents. Bioorganic & Medicinal Chemistry, 2005, 13:3513-3518.

[42]   Brown A, Brown L. Ellis D, Puhalo N, Smith CR, Wallace O, Watson L. Design and optimization of potent, selective antagonists of oxytocin. Bioorganic & Medicinal Chemistry Letters, 2008, 18: 4278-4281.

[43]   Brown A, Ellis D, Wallace O, Ralph M. Identification of amide bioisosteres of triazole Oxytocin antagonists. Bioorganic & Medicinal Chemistry Letters, 2010, 20:2224-2228.

[44]   Manikandan S. Agomelatine: a novel melatonergic antidepressant. Journal of Pharmacology & Pharmacotherapy, 2010, 1:122-123.

[45]   Millan MJ, Brocco M, Gobert A, Dekeyne, A. Anxiolytic properties of agomelatine, an antidepressant with melatoninergic and serotonergic properties: role of $5HT_{2C}$ receptor blockade. Psychopharmacology, 2005, 177:448-458.

[46]   REDDY RESEARCH FOUNDATION (India).Gaddam Om Reddy; Mamillapilli RS, Chebiyyam P. An improved process for the preparation of melatonin. IN 186858, 24 nov. 2001.

[47]   SERVIER LABORATORIES (France). Jean-Claude S, Isaac GB, Gilles T, Genevieve C, Stephane H, Gerard D. Process for the synthesis and crystalline form of agomelatine. US 7498466, 03 jan. 2008.

[48]   Knodell RG, Hall SD, Wilkinson GR, Guengerich FP. Hepatic metabolism of tolbutamide: characterization of the form of cytochrome P-450 involved in methyl hydroxylation and

relationship to *in vivo* disposition. Journal of Pharmacology and Experimental Therapeutics, 1987, 241:1112-1119.

[49]   Wermuth CG. The Practice of Medicinal Chemistry.Academic Press, 3rd edition, 2008.

[50]   Le Truong HH, Girard M, Drolet P, Grenier Y, Boucher C, Bergeron L. Spinal anesthesia: a comparison of procaine and lidocaine. Canadian Journal of Anesthesiology, 2001, 48: 470-473.

Index

A

Absorption 194
ADME/Tox 192

B

Binding affinity prediction 31
Bioisosteric replacements 17, 213

C

Chemical libraries 82
Chemical universe 64
Chemogenomic approaches 28
Consensus docking 16

D

Docking programs 92

E

Entropic contributions 37

F

Fragment-based drug design (FBDD) 14

G

Gaussian shape density 63

H

Homology modeling 9
HPC (high performance computing) 80

I

Induced fit 26

www.ingramcontent.com/pod-product-compliance
Lightning Source LLC
Chambersburg PA
CBHW050826220326

41598CB00006B/322

* 9 7 8 1 6 0 8 0 5 9 5 5 3 *